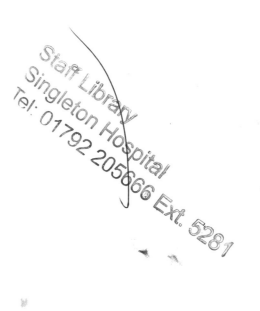

Psoriasis

Alan Menter, MD

Chair, Psoriasis Research Unit,
Baylor Research Institute
Dallas, Texas

Chief of Dermatology,
Baylor University Medical Center
Dallas, Texas

Clinical Professor of Dermatology,
University of Texas Southwestern Medical Center
Dallas, Texas

President, International Psoriasis Council (IPC)

Benjamin Stoff, MD

Chief Resident in Dermatology
Emory University School of Medicine
Atlanta, Georgia

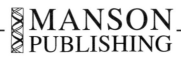

MANSON
PUBLISHING

Second Impression 2011
Copyright © 2010 Manson Publishing Ltd

ISBN: 978-1-84076-122-1

A CIP catalogue record for this book is available from the British Library.

For full details of all Manson Publishing Ltd titles please write to:
Manson Publishing Ltd, 73 Corringham Road, London NW11 7DL, UK.
Tel: +44(0)20 8905 5150
Fax: +44(0)20 8201 9233
Email: manson@mansonpublishing.com
Website: www.mansonpublishing.com

Commissioning editor: Jill Northcott
Project manager: Ayala Kingsley
Copy editor: Susie Bond
Design and illustration: Ayala Kingsley
Proof reader: John Forder
Indexer: Jill Dormon
Colour reproduction: Tenon & Polert Colour Scanning Ltd., Hong Kong
Printed by: Grafos SA, Barcelona, Spain

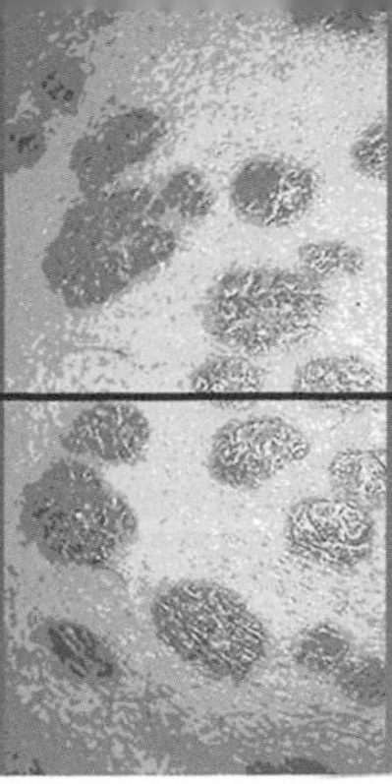

CONTENTS

Preface 5

1 HISTORY, EPIDEMIOLOGY, AND PATHOGENESIS 7

The history of psoriasis 7
Epidemiology 11
Pathogenesis: introduction 12
Histology 12
Genetics 14
Immunology 16

2 CLINICAL MANIFESTATIONS OF PSORIASIS 25

Nonpustular psoriasis (plaque type) 25
Clinical photographs
Psoriatic plaques 26
Localized nonpustular psoriasis 28
Generalized nonpustular psoriasis 43

Pustular psoriasis 26
Clinical photographs
Localized pustular psoriasis 46
Generalized pustular psoriasis 50

Other descriptors 26
Clinical photographs
Nail disease 50
Small versus large plaques 52
Stable versus unstable disease 54

3 DIFFERENTIAL DIAGNOSIS 57

Inflammatory skin disease 58
Clinical photographs
Eczema 58
Pityriasis rosea 61
Pityriasis rubra pilaris 62
Infectious disorders 64
Clinical photographs
Dermatophyte infection 64
Candida 68
Secondary syphilis 69
Neoplasms 70
Clinical photographs
Squamous cell carinoma *in situ* 70
Cutaneous T-cell lymphoma 71

4 PSORIATIC ARTHRITIS 73

General description 73
Epidemiology 73
Genetics, immunology, and pathogenesis 74
Clinical manifestations 74
Prognosis 80
Conclusion 80

5 THERAPY 81

Measuring disease 81
Therapeutic options 81
1 Topical therapy 82
2 Phototherapy and PUVA 86
3 Traditional systemic therapy 91
4 Biologics 98
Combination, rotational, and sequential regimens 108
Future directions 113

6 EFFECTS OF PSORIASIS ON
QUALITY OF LIFE   115

Physical impairment 115
Psychosocial impairment 116
Assessment tools 116
Conclusion 118

7 PSORIASIS AS A SYSTEMIC
DISEASE   119

Cardiovascular disease 119
Metabolic disorders 120
Gastrointestinal disease 121
Neurological disorders 123
Neoplastic disease 123
Psychiatric disorders 123
Mortality 124
Conclusion 124

8 APPENDIX   125

Assessment tools 125
Abbreviations 135
References 136
Clinician and patient resources 155
Index 156

ACKNOWLEDGMENTS

We wish to thank Cristina Martinez, MA, for her tireless assistance in preparing the manuscript.

PREFACE

It is with great pleasure that we present *Psoriasis*. This book is written for clinical and research-oriented dermatologists, dermatology registrars and residents, medical students, and non-physician scientists. The authors also wish to reach general practitioners, such as family and internal medicine specialists and subspecialists.

For clinical dermatologists, this book provides a concise yet thorough review of the diagnosis and treatment of the many forms of psoriatic disease, to facilitate the evaluation and care of their patients. The text also discusses current concepts in the ever-expanding field of psoriasis pathophysiology, with up-to-date graphic illustrations of key concepts. Emerging concerns, such as systemic disease associations, quality-of-life issues, and psoriatic arthritis, are also reviewed in detail.

For research-minded dermatologists, recent advances in basic science and clinical trial data are discussed. In addition, examples of well-known and validated assessment tools for psoriasis can be found in the Appendix. Readers should find helpful a chapter devoted to differential diagnosis, with juxtaposed images illustrating the main differentiating features between psoriasis and other dermatoses, common and uncommon. For interest, the authors also present a brief historical and epidemiologic discussion of the disease.

We hope that non-dermatologists, such as general and family practitioners, internal medicine specialists, rheumatologists, and specialty nurses, will also find the book valuable, as a substantial number of psoriasis patients continue to visit non-specialists for diagnosis

and treatment. New associations between psoriasis and systemic, comorbid conditions have recently been recognized and will play an important role in our further understanding of this complex disease. Knowledge of these will serve all physicians and health care professionals involved in the treatment of psoriasis, and their patients, well.

For dermatology registrars and residents, this book lays a solid foundation for learning the various aspects of psoriasis, including clinical features, differential diagnoses, laboratory findings, and therapeutic strategy. The updated sections on pathogenesis will enhance their understanding of the molecular events underlying psoriasis pathophysiology and assist in preparation for their qualifying examinations.

For medical students, this book opens a window to the intriguing world of skin disease with focus on psoriasis, a condition as pleomorphic and stigmatized as any other in dermatology. We hope to excite and encourage students to pursue further study in dermatology or even possibly a career.

For non-physician scientists, this book bridges the gap between clinical and basic science, relating the pathomechanism of disease to therapeutic targets and systemic disease associations. We hope to stimulate their interest in the investigation of inflammatory skin diseases in general and psoriasis in particular.

Ultimately, we hope the diverse content within the chapters of *Psoriasis* will elicit different responses from the variety of medical professionals whom we hope will find this book, and the various aspects of psoriasis, both interesting and enjoyable.

Alan Menter, Benjamin Stoff

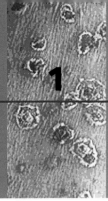

1 HISTORY, EPIDEMIOLOGY, AND PATHOGENESIS

IMAGINE a skin condition deemed so repulsive that those afflicted are forced to toll a bell announcing their presence. The diseased eat at separate tables and wear special gowns, out of fear of exposing the 'thick, prominent crust' of their skin. They are ostracized from society and, in extreme cases, even burned at the stake[1].

THE HISTORY OF PSORIASIS

The history of the skin disease recognized today as psoriasis is intertwined with other devastating conditions similar in appearance, and beset with social stigma (*Table 1*, p.9). Psoriasis shares much of its ancient history with leprosy. Various Biblical references to 'leprosy', for instance, more likely represent psoriasis. In the *Book of Kings*, the description of 'Naaman's leprosy' as 'white as snow' has led many to consider this one of the first references to the silvery scale of psoriasis[2]. Hippocrates, father of western medicine, described a series of scaling exanthems grouped under the heading '*lopoi*,' Greek for epidermis[2], which likely included both psoriasis and leprosy.

Most agree, however, that the first clinical description of psoriasis derives from Aurelius Celsus (25 BC–AD 45), in his work *De re medica*. His account of impetigo as 'having various figures ... [and] scales [that] fall off from the surface of the skin' is one such description[3]. The term 'psoriasis,' derived from the Greek '*psora*' (itch), was first used by Galen (AD 133–200). Ironically, the dermatological entity he describes as 'psoriasis,' a pruritic eruption on the eyelids and scrotum, seems more consistent with seborrheic dermatitis[4].

Associating the distinctive scaling eruption with the term 'psoriasis' was a task left for scientists of the modern era. The first in a long line of European dermatologists charged with making that association was Robert Willan (1757–1812) (**1**). In 1808, Willan

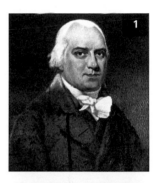

1 Robert Willan. Regarded as the founder of the field of dermatology, Willan defined psoriasis as an individual disease.

2 Ferdinand Hebra. Another forefather of dermatology, Hebra lobbied to adopt the term 'psoriasis' for the scaling skin condition.

published the first color plates of a scaling skin disease described, in his words, as 'the scaly psora by a distinct appellation; for this purpose, the term psoriasis.' However, he favored 'lepra' as the official name of the disease entity[5]. His descriptions of 'lepra' are vivid and distinct from leprosy: 'they retain a circular or oval form, and are covered with dry scales, and surrounded by a red border. Scales accumulate on them, so as to form thick crust...'

Continuing the debate over nomenclature, Ferdinand Hebra (1816–1880) (**2**), a renowned Austrian dermatologist, moved to eliminate the term 'lepra,' in favor of 'psoriasis'[6]. Others, such as Milton, disagreed fervently. 'The sooner the word psoriasis is omitted, the better. I would suggest entire expulsion of psoriasis...'[7].

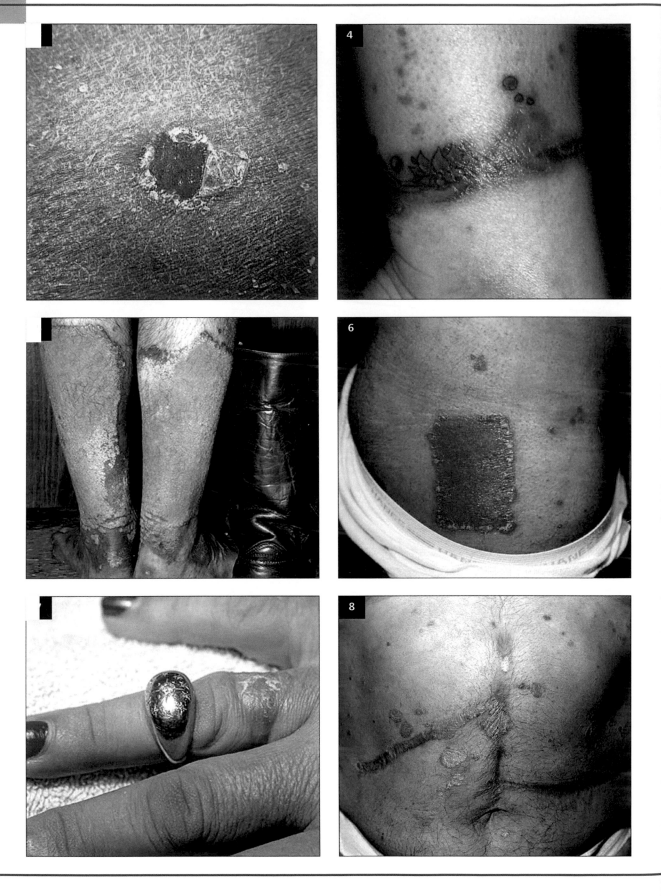

3 Auspitz sign. Removal of scale leads to pinpoint hemorrhages throughout the lesion. This corresponds to damage of dilated vessels in the superficial dermis.

4–8 Koebner phenomenon. First described by Heinrich Koebner, the development of skin lesions in areas of trauma has become known as the 'Koebner phenomenon'. This feature is characteristic of, although not specific for, psoriasis.

9 William Goeckerman. Pioneer of tar and ultraviolet light combination therapy.

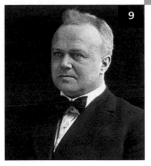

460 BC – 377 BC
Hippocrates describes scaling diseases of skin under heading 'lopoi'.

25 BC – AD 45
Celsus writes De re Medica describing the scales of 'impetigo,' likely representing psoriasis. Credited with first clinical description of psoriasis.

AD 133–200
Galen coins the term 'psoriasis,' likely in reference to seborrheic dermatitis.

1808
Robert Willan releases first color plates of psoriasis. He favors the term 'lepra.'

1868
Ferdinand Hebra argues to adopt term 'psoriasis.'

1872
Heinrich Koebner describes development of psoriatic lesions at sites of injury to skin.

1885
Heinrich Auspitz describes the pinpoint bleeding that occurs when a psoriatic scale is removed.

1898
W.J. Munro publishes first descriptions of psoriasis histology.

1910
Leo Von Zumbusch depicts a severe, pustular variant of psoriasis.

1925
William Goeckerman creates a new treatment regimen, utilizing combinations of tar and ultraviolet light.

1926
D.L. Woronoff identifies the ring of paler skin surrounding a psoriatic plaque.

1971
Methotrexate approved by the Food and Drug Administration of the United States for treatment of psoriasis.

1974
John Parrish and others publish report on combination of ultraviolet light with psoralens (PUVA) for treatment of psoriasis.

2003
First biologic, alefacept, approved by the Food and Drug Administration of the United States for moderate-to-severe psoriasis.

Over the next century, characteristics of psoriasis were described by scientists whose names would be for ever linked to the disease. Heinrich Auspitz (1835–1886), a disciple of Hebra, recognized that pinpoint bleeding occurred with the removal of scale, an entity now known as 'Auspitz sign' (3)[8]. In 1872, Heinrich Koebner described a puzzling phenomenon in which areas of recent skin trauma develop lesions of psoriasis[9]. In an address to the Silesian Society for National Culture on the cause of psoriasis, Dr Koebner recounts the development of psoriatic lesions in areas of skin traumatized by a horse bite and a tattoo (4–8).

The histology of psoriasis was also under investigation. The Australian pathologist W.J. Munro (1838–1908) noted aggregates of neutrophils within the stratum corneum of psoriatic plaques[10]. Today, these microabscesses, which carry Munro's name, are considered one of the defining histological characteristics of psoriasis.

There have also been landmarks in the treatment of psoriasis. In the 1920s, a combined therapy of coal tar application and UVB exposure, using hot quartz mercury vapor lamps, was instituted by William Goeckerman (9) at the Mayo clinic, to treat generalized psoriasis. A modified version of this treatment is still used today in specialty day-care psoriasis clinics.

Table 1 Timeline of the history of psoriasis.
Descriptions of psoriasis extend to antiquity, while scientific study of the disease began shortly after the turn of the nineteenth century.

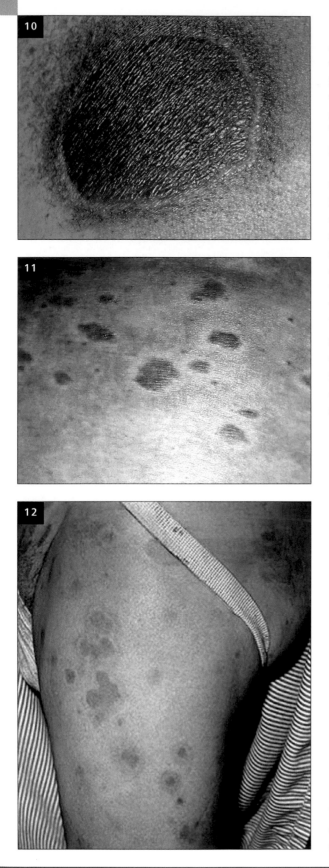

Around the same time, novel characteristics of the disease were being described. In 1910, the German Leo von Zumbusch (1874–1940) noted a severe, transient form of the disease, in which plaques were 'studded with pustules… [and] accompanied by fever and signs of toxicity'[11]. Soon after, the Russian dermatologist D.L. Woronoff gave his name to the ring of pallor surrounding a clearing psoriatic plaque (**10–12**)[12].

Historical trends in psoriasis provide insight into the challenges facing researchers and clinicians today. Over its 2000-year history, the many clinical manifestations of psoriasis have led to confusion over its identity as a distinct disease. This protean quality continues to challenge modern disease experts, who grapple with establishing a classification of psoriasis based on phenotype[13]. Thousands of years ago, societal prejudices led those affected by psoriasis to be outcast and tortured. Today psoriatics face problems with self-image, relationships, employment, ostracism, and other measures of quality of life. Current and future generations of researchers, like the forefathers of psoriasis, hope to continue advancing our understanding, and ultimately societal tolerance, of this devastating disease.

10–12 Woronoff's ring. The distinctive rim of blanching encasing a psoriatic plaque, named after the famed Russian dermatologist D.L. Woronoff.

EPIDEMIOLOGY

The study of population-based trends in psoriasis challenges epidemiologists. Several vital questions arise. What defines a case of psoriasis? What features distinguish mild from moderate-to-severe disease? What methods have been used to evaluate trends in the disease and which is best? Finally, given the great variety in case definition and methodology, how accurately can comparisons between populations be made?

Unfortunately, many of these questions remain unanswered. Nevertheless, scientists have undertaken the monumental task of assessing the epidemiology of psoriasis. Although not always uniform in approach, these works demonstrate that many aspects of the disease vary widely across different populations.

Incidence and prevalence

According to a recent international consortium, psoriasis affects up to 2% of the world's population, approximately 125 million people[14]. Despite these impressive estimates, the incidence rate (i.e. number of cases of disease per unit time) of psoriasis remains low. In one of the few studies designed to assess incidence, researchers found a rate of roughly 60 cases per 100,000 people per year[15], based on 132 newly diagnosed cases of psoriasis in Caucasians over a 4-year period at the Mayo Clinic in Rochester, Minnesota. Clearly, studies assessing more diverse populations over wider geographical areas are needed to better characterize the true incidence of disease.

As with many diseases in which onset occurs at a relatively young age and for which there is no cure, prevalence (i.e. total number of cases in a given population) can be high, despite a low incidence rate. In the UK, for instance, a recent, population-based study of 7.5 million people estimates the prevalence of psoriasis to be 1.5%[16]. This finding approximates prevalence rates in similar British populations calculated by smaller studies, which ranged from 1.58 to 2%[17,18]. In the USA, scientists estimate that psoriasis affects 7 million people[19]. Two population-based studies of Americans carried out recently reveal prevalences of 2.5–2.6%[20,21]. Interestingly, relatively fewer African-Americans appear to be affected, with recent data estimating a prevalence of 1.3%, approximately half that of Caucasians[21]. This finding is consistent with work involving native Africans, demonstrating a mere 0.8% of Nigerians of the Guinea Savanah region affected[22].

Race and ethnicity

Dramatic differences exist between other ethnicities as well. Among 25,000 native South Americans, psoriasis was undetectable[23]. The disease was also nonexistent in a population from Samoa[24]. By contrast, select populations in the Arctic maintain a disease prevalence of 12%, the highest in the world[24]. The disease appears to be relatively uncommon in Asians, with a mere 0.3% affected among a population in China[25] and 0.8% in India[26].

Gender

Like race, gender influences epidemiological trends in psoriasis. According to data from the United Kingdom, the mean age range of onset in females is significantly lower than in males, 5–9 years of age compared to 15–19, respectively[27]. In adulthood, gender prevalence equalizes[26,28]. As the population ages, data suggest that disease rates among genders may actually reverse relative to early life. According to a study of diagnostic coding data among patients older than 55 years, more males made visits to dermatologists for psoriasis than females[29]. Clearly, using clinic visits as a surrogate for prevalence is controversial. The need remains for population-based studies of psoriasis in the elderly.

Age

Groundbreaking work on age-related trends in psoriasis demonstrates a bimodal distribution[30]. Populations constituting each peak seem to have distinct genetic and phenotypic associations, leading to the population represented by the first peak to be named 'type I' psoriatics and the second 'type II.' The type I peak, comprising roughly 75% of patients with psoriasis, occurs before the age of 40. Type I patients are more likely to have first-degree relatives affected with the disease. The peak for type II psoriatics is 55–60 years of age.

Geography

The geographical distribution of psoriasis provides insight into potential factors that modify disease (*Table 2*). One such factor seems to be latitude, as sites farther from the equator maintain higher prevalence of disease than those closer. Data from the northern hemisphere (Scandinavia) and southern hemisphere (Australia) demonstrate this phenomenon, leading researchers to speculate that the effect may be mediated by differences in exposure to the ultraviolet wavelengths of sunlight[31–33].

Table 2 Prevalence of psoriasis.

[*Adapted from Farber and Nall[24] and Camp[26] with most recent data from the UK/US*]

Country / region	Population queried	Prevalence (%)
United Kingdom	7,500,000	1.5
United States (Caucasian)	21,921	2.5
United States (African–American)	2,443	1.3
Norway	10,576	1.4
Sweden	159,200	2.3
Italy	3,660	3.1
Croatia	8,416	1.5
Australia	10,037	2.3
Faroe Islands	10,984	2.8
India	20,000	0.8
China	670,000	0.3
Arctic – Kazach'ye	N/A*	11.8
South America – indigenous	25,000	0
Samoa	12,569	0

*N/A – Population not given

PATHOGENESIS: INTRODUCTION

A complex interplay between genetics and immunology culminates in the characteristic clinical and histological features of psoriasis. In predisposed individuals, a host of antigens, mostly unknown, trigger an insidious, self-perpetuating cycle of inflammation and resultant epidermal hyperproliferation. Constituents of the innate and adaptive (acquired) immune systems instigate and orchestrate this process. The two systems interface as the dendritic cell couples with the T cell, resulting in a release of signaling proteins, the cytokines. These messengers, in turn, fuel both systems, further driving the dysregulated inflammation.

Cytokines also affect keratinocytes, resulting in the abnormal epidermal growth and maturation indicative of psoriasis. Moreover, it appears that cytokines stimulate an assembly of inflammatory gene products within the keratinocyte itself, inviting more immune cells into the skin and further perpetuating the inflammatory milieu. In such a way, these simple messengers turn the target of the disease process, the keratinocyte, into a co-conspirator.

HISTOLOGY

The complexity that characterizes so many aspects of psoriasis also applies to its histology (**13–15**). Nonetheless, defining microscopic features exist, clearly visible in small, untreated lesions and at the periphery of enlarging plaques[34]. As discussed in the following chapter, these sites represent active or progressive disease, in comparison with 'stable' lesions that are static or shrinking[35,36]. However, it should be noted that despite its characteristic appearance, the histology of psoriasis may mimic a number of other dermatoses, as well as fungal or yeast infections, which must be excluded with appropriate histologic staining.

Dermis

In an unstable lesion, dilated blood vessels wind throughout the superficial dermis and proliferate. As a basic science corollary to this finding, researchers have demonstrated higher levels of the angiogenic polypeptide vascular endothelial growth factor (VEGF) in active psoriatic skin compared to normal skin[37]. Others have shown that serum levels of VEGF may correspond with extent of skin disease[38] and that upregulation of VEGF leads to psoriasiform lesions in experimental mice[39].

A collection of inflammatory cells, composed mostly of lymphocytes, infiltrates the dermis of actively diseased skin. CD4[+] T cells, natural killer T cells, and dendritic cells predominate in the dermal infiltrate, likely the result of upregulation of adhesion molecules ICAM-1 and E-selectin in dermal capillaries[40]. A unique type of surface peptide, the cutaneous lymphocyte antigen (CLA), also homes T cells to inflamed skin[41]. Edema of the dermal papillae is a common but non-specific finding.

Stable lesions also demonstrate extensive, tortuous blood vessels in the dermis. Distinct from those in unstable skin, however, these vessels extend high into papillae. This histological description corresponds to the clinical finding of pinpoint bleeding when scale is removed, known as 'Auspitz sign.' The lymphocytic infiltrate is present but less pronounced.

Epidermis

The most characteristic features of psoriasis histology lie in the epidermis. The rapid proliferation of immature keratinocytes, at rates seven times normal, exceeds terminal differentiation. Retention of keratinocyte nuclei in the stratum corneum results in a phenomenon known as parakeratosis (**13**). Whereas CD4[+] T cells and natural killer T cells predominate in the dermis, neutrophils, and, to a lesser extent, CD8[+] T cells prevail in the epidermis. Indeed, a surface protein on CD8[+] T cells, known as integrin, binds to the molecule E-cadherin on intercellular adhesion complexes in the epidermis called desmosomes[42].

Neutrophils accumulate in the stratum corneum, forming Munro microabscesses (**14**), a finding characteristic of psoriasis[34]. In stable lesions, classic psoriasiform hyperplasia evolves, with nearly uniform elongation and, occasionally, coalescence of rete ridges. Interestingly, inflammatory cell infiltration appears to precede hyperplasia[43]. Munro microabscesses may be seen in stable lesions, although much less commonly than in unstable lesions.

The pustular variant of active psoriasis demonstrates even more prominent aggregates of neutrophils infiltrating the epidermis. Intercellular edema (spongiosis) and retention of nuclei in the stratum corneum (parakeratosis) are often present. Neutrophilic foci often coalesce in the stratum spinosum to form the characteristic spongiform pustules of Kogoj (**15**).

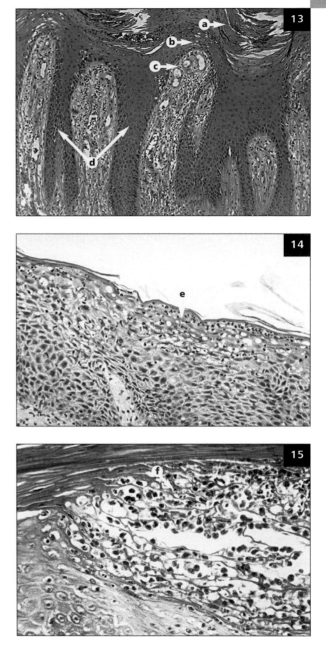

13–15 Characteristic dermapathological features:
a) **Confluent parakeratosis**
b) **Thinning of suprapapillary portion of epidermis**
c) **Edema of papilla with dilated superficial blood vessels**
d) **Regular elongation of rete ridges**
e) **Munro microabscesses**
f) **Spongiform pustules of Kogoj.**

Other characteristic histologic findings in the epidermis include attenuation of the granular layer and thinning of the epidermis overlying the dermal papillae.

GENETICS

The contribution of genes to the development of psoriasis is puzzling, but nonetheless significant. The incidence of disease, for example, increases by 30% in first-degree relatives of those affected compared to the general population[44]. Furthermore, monozygotic twins of psoriasis sufferers are two- to three-fold more likely to develop the disease than dizygotic twins[45]. Epidemiological research reveals no consistent pattern of inheritance. While autosomal recessive transmission has been demonstrated in selected families, the prevailing theory suggests autosomal dominant transmission with variable penetrance.

Decoding of the human genome has permitted extensive searches for genetic loci conferring risk of developing psoriasis (16, **Table 3**). In many cases, linkage scans have involved families with more than two affected members. As many as 19 distinct loci confer susceptibility[46]. Of these, nine have been repeatedly associated with the psoriasis phenotype, PSORSI-IX[47]. Only those maintaining the most robust associations will be discussed here.

Chromosome

Microscopic unit composed of genetic information in the form of DNA. Each chromosome is separated into a long arm ('q') and short arm ('p') by a constricting band known as the centromere.

Genes

Segments of DNA that contribute to phenotype or function.

Locus (pl. loci)

Place occupied by one or more genes on a chromosome.

Nucleotide

Fundamental unit of DNA, made up of a base (adenine, guanine, thymine, or cytosine), as well as a phosphate and sugar group.

Single nucleotide polymorphism (SNP)

An individual base within a sequence of DNA that differs from what is usually found at that position. SNPs may cause disease or form a normal variant. They are critical in conducting linkage analysis.

Linkage analysis

A complex process by which genetic loci that harbor susceptibility to disease may be identified. Traditionally, the total genetic composition, or genome, of affected sibling pairs is scanned. Genetic markers, often SNPs, are detected. If any of these markers occur at rates greater than 50% – the expected concurrence rate with sibling pairs –they may confer susceptibility to disease.

Major histocompatibility complex (MHC)

A collection of genes located on the short arm of chromosome 6 involved with the presentation of units of immunologic material – known as antigens – to T cells.

Human leukocyte antigen (HLA)

A gene or locus within the MHC.

Table 3 **Key terms in genetics.**

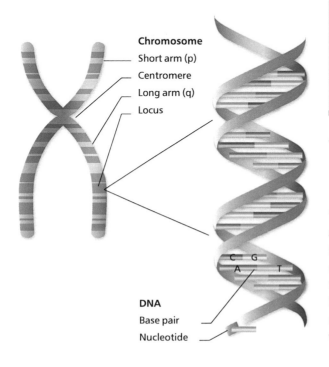

Chromosome
Short arm (p)
Centromere
Long arm (q)
Locus

DNA
Base pair
Nucleotide

C G
A T

16 Genetic loci. In humans, two pairs of 23 chromosomes are found in the nucleus of cells. Fixed positions on the chromosomes, known as loci, may be occupied by one or more genes – a specific sequence of nucleotides within the DNA molecule – that encode for particular proteins. DNA nucleotides bind across the molecule in base pairs comprising adenine (A) with thymine (T), and cytosine (C) with guanine (G).

6p21

MHC locus — p   q

Chromosome 6

HLA-C   Genes within the MHC   CCHCR   CSDN

PSORS1 (6p21)

In a disease characterized by aberrant immunity, it follows that the most significant genetic contributor described to date lies in the locus encoding the major histocompatibility complex (MHC), found on the short arm of chromosome 6 (6p21) (17). Indeed, geneticists speculate that this single site composed of fewer than 10 genes accounts for up to 50% of the heritability of psoriasis[48]. A recent, genome-wide association study confirms the significance of this locus[49]. Of over 300,000 single nucleotide polymorphisms (SNPs) typed in 223 cases of psoriasis, the nine SNPs most closely linked with disease were detected at the MHC.

The human leukocyte antigen (HLA) type 1 allele, HLA-Cw6, has demonstrated association time and again with classic, plaque-type psoriasis, but interestingly not with phenotypic variants such as palmoplantar and late-onset disease (type II, see Chapter 4, Clinical manifestations of psoriasis)[50]. The allele was found in over 50% of northern European psoriatics compared to just 7.4% of controls[51]. Puzzlingly, data suggest that only 20% of patients with psoriatic arthritis carry the allele, leading researchers to question the association of psoriatic arthritis (PsA) with the MHC locus[52]. In the genome-wide study cited above, however, SNPs from the MHC outside the allele encoding HLA-Cw6 did indeed associate strongly with PsA.

No single gene mutation leads to the psoriasis phenotype. However, several genes within the MHC locus maintain greater expression in affected skin compared to normal skin. The protein product coiled-coil α-helical rod protein 1 (CCHCR-1) results from one of these genes. The precise function of CCHCR-1 remains unclear, but lesser expression in sites of avid proliferation of keratinocytes suggests that the protein may be a negative regulator of growth[46]. Another gene product, corneodesmosin (CDSN), is overproduced in the stratum corneum of psoriatic skin[53]; the molecule promotes intercellular adhesion. Thus, scientists speculate

17 Chromosome 6 and the PSORS 1. Multiple loci within the MHC on chromosome 6 have been linked to the psoriasis phenotype, including CCHCR-1 and CDSN.

that its abundance in the epidermis of diseased skin leads to the characteristic deficiency of desquamation associated with psoriasis[46].

PSORS2 (17q25)

This was the first gene linked to psoriasis and is present on the distal portion of the long arm of chromosome 17[54-56]. Two regions within this locus have received special attention. The product of one region, the regulatory associated protein of mammalian target of rapamycin (RAPTOR), purportedly functions through inhibition of a cellular growth factor found in an array of tissues, including psoriatic skin[46]. As the name implies, MTOR, the serine-threonine kinase regulated by RAPTOR, is the target of immunomodulatory drugs rapamycin and tacrolimus. Sites of genetic variation within the RAPTOR gene associated with disease phenotype are most likely involved in the regulation of gene expression, occurring upstream of regions encoding the protein.

The other region of interest in PSORS2 contains two genes harboring risk for psoriasis. The product of one gene, solute-carrier family 9, isoform 3, regulator 1 (SLC9A3R1 or NHERF1), promotes T cell activation through the formation of a highly complex tether between the T cell and antigen presenting cell, known as the immunological synapse[46,57,58]. The function of the second gene, N-acetyltransferase 9 (NAT9), is unknown. Between these two genes, geneticists have also discovered a polymorphism for the binding site of a transcription factor RUNX1, which independently confers risk for psoriasis[55], as well as systemic lupus erythematosus and rheumatoid arthritis.

PSORS4 (1q21)

Aberrant keratinocyte differentiation, central to psoriasis scaling, undoubtedly stems from genetic abnormalities. Scientists in Italy and the United States have discovered an association between the psoriasis phenotype and a unique assemblage of genes on chromosome 1, known collectively as PSORS4[49,59,60]. The locus, also known as the epidermal differentiation complex, contains several genes that encode proteins vital to the formation of a lipid–protein envelope during the final stages of development of the epidermis[46,49,61,62,].

PSORS5 (3q21)

The remaining genetic loci linked to the psoriasis phenotype are even more puzzling to researchers. Among the cluster of genes on the long arm of chromosome 3 known as PSORS5, for example, resides SCL12A8, which encodes the transporter of an as yet undescribed cation[63,64]. SCL12A8 belongs to a family of transporter genes, many of which appear to be altered in autoimmune diseases such as Crohn's disease and rheumatoid arthritis[46].

Table 4 Susceptibility loci for psoriasis.

[Adapted from Duffin KC, Chandran V, Gladman DD, et al. Genetics of Psoriasis and Psoriatic Arthritis: Update and Future Direction. Journal of Rheumatology 2008; 35: 1449–1453]

Locus	Region	Candidate gene/Product
PSORS1	6p21	HLA-Cw6, CDSN, CCHCR1 [HCR, HERV-K, HCG2, 7PS04S1C3, POU5F1, TCF19, LMP, SEEK1, SPR1]
PSORS2	17q25	RAPTOR, SLC9A3R1, NAT9, RUNX1, [TBCD]
PSORS3	3q	IRF-2
PSORS4	1q21	Epidermal Differentiation Complex, [Loricrin, Filaggrin, Pglyrp3]
PSORS5	3q21	SLC12A8, [Cystatin A, Zn Finger protein 148]
PSORS6	19p13	[JunB]
PSORS7	1p	[PTPN22], IL-23R
PSORS8	16q	[CX3CL1, CX3R1], NOD2/CARD15
PSORS9	4q31	IL-15
PSORS10	18p11	unknown

Other PSORS loci

A wide range of additional loci, including PSORS3 and PSORS 6–10, have been also shown to confer risk for the psoriasis phenotype (**Table 4**). The contribution of these loci are probably less meaningful than their more well-established counterparts, such as PSORS1 (see above). Several of these loci encode proteins that are relevant to psoriasis pathophysiology, such as a subunit of interleukin-23 (PSORS7) and interleukin-15 (PSORS 9), both cytokine promoters of cell-mediated inflammation. PSORS 3 contains interferon regulatory factor 2, IRF-2, which encodes an inhibitor of interferon α and γ expression. The locus encoding NOD2/CARD15 (PSORS 8) confers susceptibility to both psoriasis and Crohn's disease, another immune-mediated condition, increasingly seen together clinically.

IMMUNOLOGY

The revolution in psoriasis treatment brought about by the biological agents discussed in detail in Chapter 5, Therapy, has spurred interest in immunology among researchers. As a result, our knowledge of the immune basis of psoriasis has grown considerably since cyclosporin was first shown, serendipitously, to benefit psoriasis[65]. Thus far, a complex story has unraveled, involving interplay of innate and adaptive immunity. Nonetheless, several key players – including the full range of T cells and dendritic cells – orchestrate the pathogenesis of psoriasis to a greater extent than others and therefore deserve special attention.

T cells

Chief coordinators of the immune system, T cells evolve into several subtypes (**Table 5**). Of those displaying surface antigens, known as cluster of differentiation (CD), CD4 and CD8 are the most common and familiar. Put simply, CD4[+] T cells choreograph the immune response, thus the designation 'helper' T cells. In contrast, CD8[+] T cells execute the immune response, either directly through killing a targeted cell or indirectly through suppression of other immune cells. In large quantities, both types infiltrate psoriatic lesions and are highly active[66]. Other T cell variants, such as natural killer T (NKT) cells and CD4[+] T cells producing interleukin-17 (T_H17 cells), enter the fray as well. As expected, the only T cell subtype shown to be lacking in psoriasis is the regulatory type[67].

CD4$^+$ T cells

Chief coordinators of the immune response, these T cells are found predominantly in the dermis of lesions and may evolve via the T$_H$1 or T$_H$17pathway, leading to a cell-mediated, rather than antibody-mediated, immune response.

CD8$^+$ T cells

Important in targeted cell killing and suppression of other immune cells, these T cells are found in the epidermis of psoriatic lesions and have been found to play a role in cytokine trafficking.

Antigen presenting cells (APCs)

Cells which engulf, process, and present antigens to other cells. Examples of APCs include dendritic cells (both dermal and plasmacytoid) and Langerhans cells.

Cytokines

Proteins that allow local communication between cells.

Table 5 Important players in the immunology of psoriasis.

CD8$^+$ T cells

As mentioned under Histology, the composition of the T cell infiltrate in a psoriatic plaque varies according to microanatomic location. That is, CD8$^+$ T cells predominate in the epidermis, while CD4$^+$ T cells predominate in the dermis. The epidermal inflammatory infiltrate expands, in part, via adhesion molecules, called integrins, found on the surface of the T cell. Most CD8$^+$ T cells in psoriasis lesions express lymphocyte function-associated antigen 1 (LFA-1), which binds to intercellular adhesion molecules (ICAMs) on the endothelial cell surface of dermal capillaries and forms the target of the biologic drug efalizumab (see Chapter 5, Therapy)[46]. Many CD8$^+$ T cells home to the epidermis further through the binding of a different integrin to E-cadherin on the desmosome[42]. The surface of these CD8$^+$ T cells also contains receptors for distinct intercellular mediators, known as cytokines (see below). Specifically, scientists have discovered CXC-chemokine receptor 3 (CXCR3), which binds corresponding substances released by diseased keratinocytes[68]. Indeed, cytokine trafficking may be even more central to the role of CD8$^+$ cells in psoriasis than cell killing, a theory supported by the abundance of cytokines but lack of premature keratinocyte death in affected skin[46].

CD4$^+$ T cells

Invasion of CD4$^+$ T cells into the dermis marks the beginning stage of development of the psoriasis lesion[34]. Indeed, the number of CD4$^+$ T cells mirrors lesion activity clinically, falling off as the plaque stabilizes and ultimately remits. Upon activation, CD4$^+$ T cells evolve into two distinct types based on the assemblage of cytokines produced: T$_H$1 cells, which promote cell-mediated inflammation, and T$_H$2 cells, which elicit antibody-mediated inflammation. In psoriasis, the balance tips heavily in favor of the production of T$_H$1 cells resulting in rigorous cell-mediated inflammation. Cytokines produced by T$_H$1 cells include interleukin-2 (IL-2), interferon gamma (IFN-γ), and, perhaps most noteworthy, tumor necrosis factor alpha (TNF-α). Several of the biological drugs – including adalimumab, etanercept, and infliximab – target the latter (see Chapter 5, Therapy).

Other T cells

NKT cells and CD4$^+$ T cells produce interleukin-17 (T$_H$17 cells).

At the intersection of innate and adaptive immunity, the NKT cell found in psoriatic plaques maintains some markers of the T lymphocyte lineage, as well as the killer-cell immunoglobulin-like receptor (KIR) found on natural killer cells[46,69]. The precise function of the NKT cell remains uncertain; however, evidence suggests that, at the very least, the cell secretes IFN-γ, a key player in cell-mediated inflammation (see below)[70]. Some even speculate that the NKT cell, through reception of antigens such as glycolipids, may actually incite the inflammatory cascade in psoriasis[49].

Also piquing the interest of psoriasis researchers, a unique CD4$^+$ T cell has recently been found in affected skin. The cell evolves under the influence of interleukin 23 (IL-23), secreted by specialized dendritic cells (see below), and produces interleukin-17 (IL-17), leading to the designation 'T$_H$17 cell'[71]. IL-17, along with TNF-α and IFN-γ, induce keratinocytes to produce other proinflammatory cytokines, such as interleukin-8 (see below)[72]. Indeed, many scientists believe this brand of T cell, rather than the traditional T$_H$1 cell, actually drives the development of the psoriatic plaque[73]. This postulate owes in part to recent work demonstrating the development of psoriatic plaques in mice in response to the injection of IL-23, as well as impressive clinical efficacy of antibodies targeting IL-12/23. These specialized

CD4$^+$ T cells also turn out interleukin-22 (IL-22), recently implicated in psoriasiform thickening of the epidermis (see below).

Antigen-presenting cells: dendritic cells

Unable to recognize immunogenic material in native form, T cells require special presentation of antigens, as well as further stimulation, to become fully active. The task of recognizing, processing, and displaying antigenic substances in a way suitable for the T cell falls to the antigen-presenting cell (APC) (*Table 6*) (18). APCs exhibit antigenic peptides in a unique intracellular scaffold, which, upon exposure to the antigen, translocates to the cell surface bound to peptide. This scaffold derives from a highly-polymorphic gene locus, known as the major histocompatibility complex (MHC). As discussed above, the MHC, found on chromosome 6, overlaps with a well-established susceptibility locus for psoriasis, PSORS1.

18 The interplay of T-cells and antigen-presenting cells in psoriasis. Antigen-presenting cells, such as dendritic cells (DCs), mature upon exposure to antigen and begin to elicit important cytokines such as TNF-α (1). TNF-α facilitates the extravasation from the blood of circulating T cells via a sequence of interactions which includes the binding of cutaneous lymphocyte antigen 1 (CLA) with E-selectin, and leukocyte function-associated antigen 1 (LFA-1) with intercellular adhesion molecule 1 (ICAM-1) (2–4). Entering the dermis, the T cells are activated by the DCs, which present the specific antigen for a given T cell, binding multiple receptors in addition to the antigen/MHC molecule and T-cell receptor (5). Once activated, DCs and T cells produce other cytokines such as IL-12 and IL-23, and interferon gamma (IFN-γ). The cumulative effect of this cytokine milieu is the epidermal hyperproliferation characteristic of psoriasis.

[Adapted with permission from Kupper TS (2003). Immunologic targets in psoriasis. New England Journal of Medicine 349: 1987–1990]

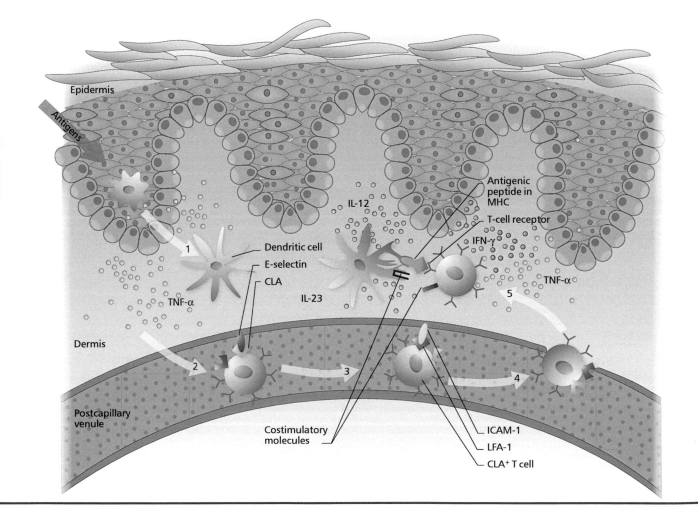

Type	Trigger
Infectious	*Streptococcus pyogenes*
	Human immunodeficiency virus (HIV)
Pharmacologic	Lithium
	Corticosteroids (upon withdrawal)
	Beta-blocking agents
	Anti-malarials
Other	Psychological stress
	Smoking (especially in palmoplantar psoriasis)
	Alcohol
	Climate (cold, lack of sunlight)

Table 6 Potential antigenic triggers of psoriasis.

Genes of the MHC encode two broad classes of molecule for the presentation of antigens. The MHC class I molecules, found on all nucleated cells, interact with $CD8^+$ T cells, whereas MHC class II molecules, found only on APCs, interact with $CD4^+$ T cells. Sentinel among the APCs, dendritic cells (DCs) are found in the skin, as well as other sites of pathogen entry such as mucosal tissue, heart, and portal area of the liver. It is the only type of APC that, upon migration to the lymph node, activates naive T cells, thereby initiating adaptive immunity[74]. During this migration, the DC matures to the form capable of activating the T cell, as demonstrated by expression of proteins CD83 and DC lysosomal-associated membrane protein (LAMP) on the cell surface[75]. In support of the general role of DCs in psoriasis, 'unstable' psoriatic lesions maintain higher numbers of activated DCs than stable or uninvolved skin[76].

Interaction between the MHC molecules, loaded with peptide on the surface of the DC, and corresponding T cell receptor (TCR) is not sufficient to activate T cells, however. Full activation requires a second signal, termed costimulation, resulting from the binding of a distinct surface protein on the DC to a receptive protein on the T cell. Immunologists suggest that a third signal, involving cytokines, determines the fate of the $CD4^+$ T cell with respect to the T_H1 versus T_H2 pathway[74].

Several types of dendritic cells exist, differentiated by unique collections of proteins on the cell surface. DCs also undergo a prescribed maturation process, from initial recognition of antigen at the site of entry to presentation to and costimulation of T cells in the lymph node. Clearly, the potential for derangement exists. Psoriasis researchers point to three types of dendritic cells – Langerhans cells, dermal DCs, and plasmacytoid Dcs – as perpetrators of psoriasis pathogenesis.

Langerhans cells ($CD1a^+$, HLA-DR$^+$)
Stellate cells of lymphoid origin, Langerhans cells are chiefly responsible for immunity in normal skin. Upon activation by exposure to antigenic substrate, these cells mature to potent stimulators of T cells and producers of cytokines (e.g. TNF-α, IL-6, IL-8, and IL-12). Evidence demonstrates a greater number of these cells in affected skin of some patients with psoriasis[77]. Recent work also reveals that transmigration of Langerhans cells from the epidermis to the lymph node is impaired in psoriasis lesions[78]. Despite their central role as bridges of innate and adaptive immunity in normal skin, Langerhans cells may not be the most important dendritic cell players in psoriasis[79].

Dermal dendritic cells (factor XIIIa$^+$, $CD11c^+$)
Another type of dendritic cell resides in the dermis, thus the name 'dermal' DC. The dermal DC derives from myeloid precursors, as indicated by expression of $CD11c^+$ on the cell surface[80]. As a pharmacologic corollary, CD11a forms the target of the biologic agent efalizumab (see Chapter 5, Therapy). Dermal DCs infiltrate involved skin to a much greater degree than normal skin[81]. They are so plentiful, in fact, that scientists estimate the population of $CD11c^+$ DCs in affected skin to equal, or even exceed, the T cell population[82].

Dermal DCs appear to play a dual role in psoriasis pathophysiology. They demonstrate markers of activation, such as CD83$^+$, suggesting the ability to stimulate T cells in a manner similar to Langerhans cells and also secrete several cytokines involved in psoriatic inflammation, such as TNF-α, inducible nitric oxide synthase (iNOS), and, to a lesser extent, IL-20 and 23[80,83].

Plasmacytoid dendritic cells (CD11c⁻, HLA-DR⁺, CD123⁺)

A unique subset of DCs – plasmacytoid dendritic cells (pDCs) – has recently been found in greater amounts in psoriasis lesions as compared to normal skin[84]. Purportedly, the binding of an as yet unspecified antigen to a toll-like receptor (TLR), harbinger of innate immunity, activates pDCs to elicit massive amounts of interferon alpha (IFN-α). This inflammatory cytokine, in turn, promotes production of T_H1 cells, ramping up inflammation and resulting in the clinical appearance of a psoriatic plaque. Indeed, activation of pDCs via one such TLR, toll-like receptor 7, by the agonist imiquimod resulted in psoriatic lesions, according to a recent study[49,85].

Groundbreaking work also implicates TLR-9 as an important stimulus for pDCs in psoriasis pathophysiology[86]. In an elegant series of experiments, the endogenous, antimicrobial peptide LL37 was found to couple with self-DNA from damaged keratinocytes in condensed structures engulfed by pDCs. These structures trigger TLR-9, subsequent release of INF, and ultimately, inflammation. This mechanism, the authors suggest, may explain how self-DNA, normally tolerated by the innate immune system, becomes a potent target in psoriasis. As damaged DNA is released during skin injury, these LL37–DNA aggregates may also explain the Koebner phenomenon.

19 Potential cytokine network in psoriasis. Upon maturation/activation, dermal and plasmacytoid DCs elicit cytokines, including IL-12 and IL-23, which stimulate evolution of T cells into T_H1 or T_H17 cells (1). These, in turn, produce IL-17, IL-22, IFN-γ, and TNF-α, which activate transcription factors, such as STAT and NF-κB, within the keratinocyte (2). This results in upregulation of pro-inflammatory genes (3), and, ultimately, growth factors including transforming growth factor alpha (TGF-α) (4).

[Adapted with permission from Lowes MA, Bowcock AM, Krueger JG (2007). Pathogenesis and therapy of psoriasis. Nature 445: 866–873]

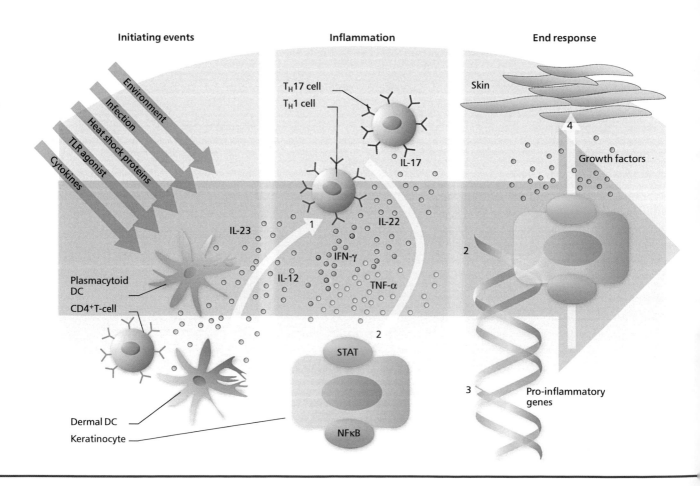

Cytokines

With greater understanding of inflammation in psoriasis, scientists have recognized the critical role of cytokines. Similar to hormones, these soluble proteins act as mediators between cells. This intercellular dialog is crucial for coordinated processes, of which inflammation is a prime example (**19**). The term 'cytokine' applies broadly to entities like interleukins, lymphokines, chemokines, and other signaling molecules, such as tumor necrosis factors and interferons.

Nearly 20 years ago, psoriasis researchers realized that a complex interplay of these molecules contributes to the development of disease[73,87]. Since then, knowledge has exploded. Now, cytokines provide not only insight into psoriasis pathophysiology but also a ready target for a new line of biological drugs that have revolutionized psoriasis treatment. These molecules have also refocused energies to determine the mechanism of action of traditional agents.

Tumor necrosis factor alpha (TNF-α)

Much of the excitement in cytokine research surrounds the 157-amino acid homotrimer TNF-α. The term 'tumor necrosis factor' derives from early experiments demonstrating activity of the peptide against malignant cells[55]. Scientists discovered that much of this effect spawned from local inflammation and, to a lesser extent, initiation of acquired immunity. General inflammatory properties of TNF-α include, for example, induction of leukocyte adhesion molecules intercellular adhesion molecule-1 (ICAM-1) and vascular adhesion molecule-1 (VCAM-1) in capillaries, allowing for influx of inflammatory cells from the bloodstream[88]. TNF-α also recruits and stimulates the activity of neutrophils, a major component of the inflammatory infiltrate in psoriasis, both directly and via stimulation of IL-8 production by monocytes[55]. TNF-α directly primes the adaptive immune system as well, through upregulation of MHC molecules on antigen-presenting cells[89] (**20**).

In psoriasis, TNF-α performs the general duties mentioned above, as well as several others vital to disease evolution. As in other sites of inflammation, TNF-α in psoriatic plaques stimulates adhesion molecules ICAM-1, VCAM-1, and E-selectin on the surface of endothelial cells in dermal capillaries[34,90]. Through the mechanisms discussed, TNF-α in active lesions also elicits neutrophils, which coalesce to form characteristic Munro microabscesses and spongiform pustules of Kogoj[34].

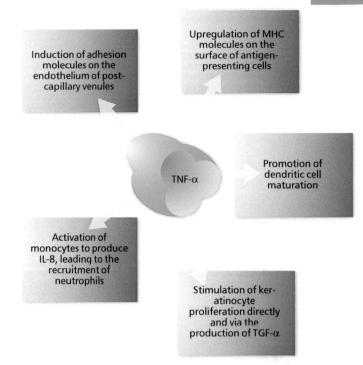

20 Inflammatory properties of TNF-α. TNF-α plays multiple roles in the inflammatory process, both directly and indirectly.

TNF-α stimulates epidermal proliferation both directly and indirectly through the induction of transforming growth factor alpha (TGF-α)[34,80]. The cytokine affects keratinocytes further through upregulation of adhesion molecule and chemokine production via recently described molecular pathways[46]. It promotes dendritic cell maturation by stimulating surface expression of CD83[+], thereby also propagating adaptive immunity[91].

A molecule so essential to psoriasis requires an army of cells to maintain its production. Cleverly, many of the cells that produce TNF-α are also stimulated by TNF-α. Thus, the intricate cycle of psoriasis pathogenesis is self-perpetuating. The dermal dendritic cell, for instance, avidly produces TNF-α[46]. In turn, TNF-α induces dendritic cell maturation. Keratinocytes demonstrate a similar give and take with TNF-α, maintaining steady production while receiving potent stimulation for the cytokine[80]. With multiple positive feedback loops at play, it is no surprise that TNF-α levels are markedly elevated in psoriatic plaques[92], as well as in the synovium of affected joints in patients with psoriatic arthritis.

The abundance and diversity of action of TNF-α in psoriasis have made it an attractive target for drug development. As described in Chapter 4, Psoriatic arthritis, this cytokine also plays a similar pathogenic role in the development of the related inflammatory arthropathy, psoriatic arthritis, further enticing pharmaceutical researchers. As mentioned above, three drugs directed at TNF-α are currently approved for psoriasis and psoriatic arthritis – adalimumab, etanercept, and infliximab – with others in this class under development. The effect of these drugs, part of a growing class known as biological agents (see Chapter 5, Therapy), on psoriasis treatment has been revolutionary.

Other cytokines

The overexpression of numerous other proinflammatory cytokines (IL-8, IL-12, IFN-γ, IL-17, IL-22, IL-23), as well as the low expression of anti-inflammatory cytokines, such as IL-10, is also typical of psoriatic skin. Cytokines direct keratinocyte hyperproliferation and the cellular composition of the inflammatory infiltrate within the plaques, involving both the innate and aquired immune systems (**21**).

Interleukin 10 (IL-10)

CD4$^+$ T cells programmed to promote antibody-mediated or humoral immunity, known as T_H2 cells, diminish the alternative T_H1 pathway with the secretion of IL-10. T_H1 diseases, however, counter by down-regulating T_H2 cytokines, including IL-10. The finding of low levels of IL-10 in psoriatic plaques, therefore, comes as no surprise[93]. Further support for a role of IL-10 stems from the discovery of a genetic linkage between the IL-10 promoter and a familial psoriasis phenotype[61]. These findings have prompted researchers to supplement psoriasis patients with IL-10 in hopes of quieting the overactive T_H1 pathway[94]. To date, results have been disappointing.

Interleukin 8 (IL-8)

In contrast to other interleukins, IL-8 is a chemotactic cytokine, attracting, rather than stimulating or suppressing, other immune cells, and so is more specifically described by the term 'chemokine'. Local neutrophils and activated T cells are drawn to sites of inflammation by following a chemokine concentration gradient towards the source of the chemokine[34], leaving the bloodstream and entering the epidermis. As expected, psoriatic lesions demonstrate markedly elevated levels of IL-8[95]. Multiple cells – keratinocytes, monocytes, and fibroblasts – produce the chemokine under the influence of other cytokines such as TNF-α[34].

Interferon gamma (IFN-γ) and interleukin-12 (IL-12)

Principle cytokines of cell-mediated immunity, IL-12 and IFN-γ serve prominent roles in psoriasis. Produced by activated T_H1 cells and dermal dendritic cells, IFN-γ signals the transcription of multiple immune-related genes in psoriasis lesions, including those encoding leukocyte adhesion molecules, cytokines, and receptors[70]. The transcription factor signal transducer and activator of transcription 1 (STAT1) likely represents the molecular liaison between IFN-γ and these genes[96,97]. From the perspective of cytokines, that is, IFN-γ may be the final common stimulus for the amplification of the T_H1 response.

To produce IFN-γ, T_H1 cells require stimulation from other cytokines. IL-12, immunologists believe, provides this stimulation[98]. Primed with antigenic peptide, APCs bound to and costimulated by T cells secrete the cytokine, propagating cell-mediated immunity. Due to heavy reliance on T_H1-mediated inflammation in psoriasis, researchers postulated that IL-12 plays a vital part in disease pathogenesis[87]. Indeed, infusion of IL-12 induces cutaneous inflammation and hyperplasia in mice[99]. Recently, however, researchers have challenged the central role of IL-12/IFN-γ in psoriasis, shifting focus to a recently described, alternative pathway (see below).

Interleukin-17 (IL-17), interleukin-22 (IL-22), and interleukin-23 (IL-23)

Foremost cytokines in this new model are IL-17, IL-23, and, most recently, IL-22[87]. Excitement began with the discovery of a unique brand of CD4$^+$ T cell, as described above, which produces IL-17[71]. This T_H17 cell is not an avid producer of IFN-γ, prohibiting traditional categorization as a T_H1 cell. Among other roles, IL-17 stimulates the production of inflammatory cytokines by macrophages and keratinocytes[72].

This perplexing T_H17 cell also produces IL-22. In recent experiments, IL-22 infusion induced epidermal hyperplasia[99]. Conversely, genetic knockout or pharmacological inhibition of IL-22 decreased epidermal thickness. Further, IL-22 may stimulate the all-important STAT pathway within keratinocytes[73,100].

To evolve into IL-17 producers, naive CD4[+] T cells require stimulation from IL-23[69]. Produced by activated dendritic cells, IL-23 permeates psoriatic skin to a much greater degree than normal skin[101]. The cytokine shares a common subunit with IL-12, a target for recent drug development (see Chapter 5, Therapy). However, IL-23 does not appear to stimulate $T_H 1$ cells to produce IFN-γ. To illustrate this, scientists recently showed that injections of IL-23 failed to produce increased levels of IFN-γ, while leading to elevated levels of IL-17 and IL-22[98]. Interestingly, the same experiment demonstrated greater epidermal hyperplasia in skin treated with IL-23 than with IL-12, suggesting that this new IL-23–IL-17 pathway may in fact play a more central role in psoriasis pathogenesis than the classic $T_H 1$ pathway. Further supporting this theory, geneticists have demonstrated significant linkage between loci encoding the IL-23 receptor and the psoriasis/PsA phenotype[49].

21 The pathogenesis of psoriasis: the interface of innate and acquired immunity. This involves a delicate balance between genetic and environmental factors as well as innate and acquired immunity. Cytokines produced by keratinocytes activate both the innate (neutrophils and dendritic cells) and acquired (T cells and NK T cells) immune systems (1, 2). These systems are primed by environmental factors such as activators (agonists) of toll-like receptors (TLRs) and bacterial antigens. Ultimately, genetic factors lead to dysregulated production of cytokines by both systems, which stimulate aberrant terminal differentiation of keratinocytes. The two systems interface at the interaction of the T cell and mature dendritic cell (3).

[Adapted with permission from Lowes et al (2007). Pathogenesis and therapy of psoriasis. Nature 445: 866–873]

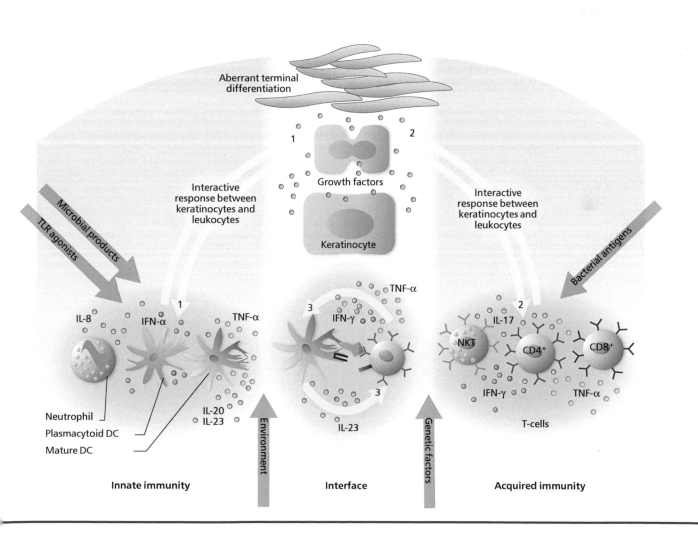

Other cells: neutrophils, monocytes, and macrophages

Neutrophils

Polymorphonuclear cells, or neutrophils, comprise several characteristic features of psoriasis histology. A variety of signaling factors call neutrophils to action in psoriasis lesions, including IL-8, complement split product 5a, and leukotriene B4[91]. Despite the classic microscopic appearance, neutrophils are not found in consistently large quantities across biopsy specimens of active lesions from different patients with classic psoriasis vulgaris[84].

Macrophages and monocytes

Vital participants in cellular immunity, monocytes and macrophages assume a secondary role in psoriasis pathophysiology. They penetrate basement membrane, stimulating keratinocyte growth by secreting IL-6, among other cytokines[34]. With appropriate stimulation, these cells also evolve into dermal dendritic cells, which retain the surface CD11a vestige [84].

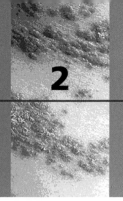
2 CLINICAL MANIFESTATIONS OF PSORIASIS

PSORIASIS is extremely polymorphic. From a few subtle pits in the nail plate to discrete small plaques to full-blown erythroderma, the disease defies simple classification. Consequently, a formal taxonomy of psoriasis was not available for the first 200 years of its life as an entity of scientific study. A myriad of problems ensued. What defined a case of psoriasis? If distinct subtypes existed, were there differences in epidemiologic trends, genetic bases, and natural histories among the various types? Perhaps most relevant to recent advances in psoriasis treatment, how does the range of phenotypes respond to new therapies and are data from different trials comparable?

In 2006, experts in the field responded with a new proposal for classification of psoriasis phenotypes[1]. This chapter follows the categorization set out in their work, which organizes types based on presence or absence of pustules and localized or generalized anatomical distribution, as well as other miscellaneous descriptors, such as nail disease.

Nonpustular psoriasis: psoriatic plaques

22 Classic discoid plaques. Note the silvery scale, sharp circumscription, and accentuated border.

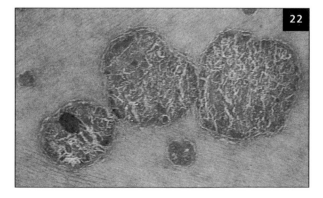

22

NONPUSTULAR PSORIASIS (PLAQUE TYPE)

The most common expression of psoriatic skin disease, plaque-type psoriasis, comprises 90% of cases[2]. The classic oval plaque, erythematous with silvery scale, characterizes this form (**22**). Well-circumscribed lesions expand centrifugally, with an active, evolving edge[3]. Experts observe that, as plaques grow, central clearing may give the lesion an annular rather than discoid appearance. Plaques can be small or large, discrete or confluent, isolated or disseminated (**23–28**, p. 27).

Localized nonpustular psoriasis

The classic plaques of psoriasis form on the trunk and limbs. The preferred sites include the well-known extensor surfaces of the knees and elbows, but also the lower back, flanks, and umbilicus (**29–70**, pp. 28–35).

Plaque-type psoriasis favors other sites as well. Lesions may assume a seborrheic distribution, a condition known as 'sebo-psoriasis.' Plaques form in the nasolabial folds, cheeks, scalp and scalp line, eyebrows, intermammary and interscapular areas. In this subtype, lesions are thinner (often less than 0.75 mm) and scales are more 'waxy' than the classic form. Indeed, the clinician may distinguish sebo-psoriasis from seborrheic dermatitis only by the presence of psoriasis elsewhere, by family history of psoriasis, and/or by the presence of psoriatic arthritis (**71–74**, p. 36).

A variant of plaque-type psoriasis affects flexural and intertriginous areas (**75–86**, pp. 37, 38). Involved sites include axillae, inguinal folds, gluteal cleft, and inframammary region. Lesions are thin, as in sebo-psoriasis, but less scaly and more erythematous. Friction can give rise to maceration and, not uncommonly, secondary candidiasis.

Psoriasis invariably targets the scalp (**87–96**, pp.39, 40), frequently as a first manifestation of the disease. Lesions may be localized or diffuse, thick or thin. Unlike psoriasis elsewhere, scalp disease tends to be asymmetric, possibly due to rubbing, scratching, or picking of lesions in this area by the patient. Lesions rarely extend beyond one inch distally from the scalp line and frequently favor the posterior auricular area. Other areas bearing hair may be affected.

An interesting variant of localized, nonpustular psoriasis affects the palms and soles. In contrast to typical plaques, borders are diffuse and more erythematous. Secondary fissuring may be prominent. Lesions may be discrete or confluent, and may extend distally along the fingers (**97–108**, pp. 40–42).

Generalized nonpustular psoriasis

Diffuse psoriasis may represent widespread trunk and limb disease or unique subtypes that lack a localized form. Guttate psoriasis manifests with small (less than 1 cm), scaly papules typically spread over the trunk (**109–114**, p.43). These salmon-pink lesions purportedly resemble raindrops, as *gutta* is Latin for 'drop.' Classically, lesions develop *de novo* in young people after an infection with streptococcus. Progression occurs over a 3-month period, as the eruption develops in the first month, persists over the second, and resolves in the third. Approximately one-third of those affected develop chronic, plaque-type psoriasis[1]. A guttate flare may also occur in patients with plaque-type psoriasis, either after a streptococcal infection or as part of a flare of the disease.

In its most severe form, psoriasis produces erythroderma (**115–122**, pp. 44, 45), affecting major portions of the body's surface area. The condition typically arises in patients with chronic psoriasis after withdrawal of oral corticosteroids, abrupt cessation of standard treatments, such as methotrexate and phototherapy, burns, or infections. In rare cases, erythroderma presents *de novo*. Generalized erythema and exfoliation may lead to life-threatening volume depletion, electrolyte disturbances, high output heart failure, and even death.

Nonpustular psoriasis: psoriatic plaques
23–28 Morphology and distribution.

PUSTULAR PSORIASIS

Localized pustular psoriasis

Crops of monomorphic, sterile pustules characterize pustular psoriasis (**123–138**, pp.46–48). In the limited form of the disease, two puzzling subtypes exist. Indeed, researchers have demonstrated that at least one of these subtypes, palmoplantar pustular psoriasis, maintains a genetic and epidemiologic identity distinct from plaque-type psoriasis[4,5]. Only 20% of patients with palmoplantar pustular psoriasis demonstrate psoriasis elsewhere[1]. The variant is more common in women and smokers.

Another form of localized pustular psoriasis, acrodermatitis continua of Hallopeau (**139–146**, p. 49), affects the distal portions of the fingers and toes with extensive adjacent nail dystrophy, paronychial erythema and edema. Other types of psoriasis, pustular palmoplantar, and/or plaque-type, may exist concomitantly.

Generalized pustular psoriasis

The striking generalized pustular psoriasis (**147, 148**, p. 50), also known as 'von Zumbusch type' after the German dermatologist who described the condition, may develop in the setting of longstanding or new cases of psoriasis. Signs of systemic toxicity, such as lower-leg edema, fever, leukocytosis, and myalgias, accompany this variant. As with erythrodermic psoriasis, withdrawal of glucocorticoids is a classic trigger[6].

OTHER DESCRIPTORS

Nail disease

Often overlooked, nail disease affects 40–50% of psoriatics[1]. Nail disease varies significantly in appearance; however, any type may predict the presence of psoriatic arthritis in adjacent joints[7]. Small indentations, or pits, in the nail plate are commonly present, secondary to small foci of parakeratosis in the nail matrix (**149–152**, p. 50)[8]. Although not specific, disorganized pits numbering more than 20 may distinguish psoriasis from other dermatoses associated with pitting, such as alopecia areata, in which pits are more uniform[9].

Another common but nonspecific manifestation of nail psoriasis, onycholysis, occurs as the distal nail plate separates from the bed (**153–156**, p. 51).

Translucent subungual macules with a brownish hue, known as 'oil drops,' also characterize the nail disease of psoriasis (**157, 158**, p. 51).

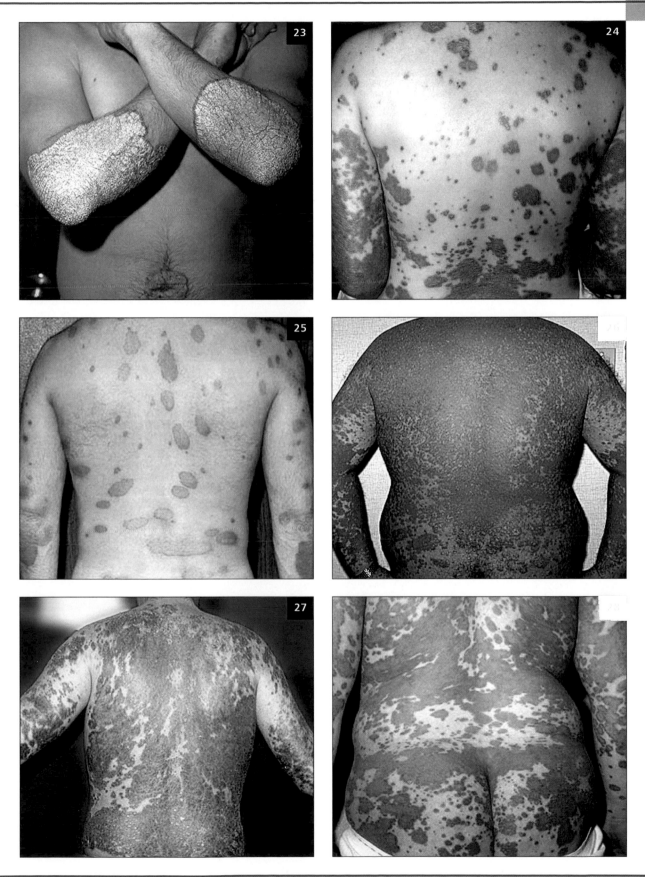

Accumulation of keratotic debris causes subungual hyperkeratosis (**159, 160**, p. 51). Although the nail plate appears thickened, the condition actually results from abnormal maturation of the nail bed.

Small versus large plaques

It is appropriate to distinguish small plaques (<3 cm) (**161–166**, p. 52) from large plaques (>3 cm) (**167–171**, p. 53). Follicular psoriasis, a rare form of small plaque disease, is depicted in **161** and **162**.

Stable versus unstable disease

The state of disease is also described as stable or unstable. Expansion of pre-existing psoriasis or development of new lesions defines unstable disease (**172–183**, pp. 54–56). Static or remitting disease is considered stable, although involvement may still be extensive. The common Koebner phenomenon, in which lesions develop at sites of skin injury, is depicted in **181–183**.

PASI

The Psoriasis Area and Severity Index (PASI) is a standardized, validated tool used to assess severity of disease (see Appendix). Although rarely used in clinical practice, PASI is a hallmark of clinical trials. The instrument quantifies induration, erythema, scale, and extent of body surface area (BSA) involvement in four body regions – head and neck, trunk, upper extremities, and lower extremities (including buttocks). Reduction in PASI score corresponds to improvement in disease. The PASI has evolved into the primary measuring tool of drug efficacy, with a PASI 75 (i.e. 75% reduction in score) traditionally constituting a significant response to therapy[10–12]. Some disease experts suggest, however, that PASI 50 may serve as a meaningful target for the effectiveness of therapy[13]. This assertion is debatable, as many patients express dissatisfaction with responses falling short of PASI 75. In addition, PASI 90, near complete clearing of disease, may become a meaningful parameter with the emergence of the newer anti-IL-12/23 biologic drugs (see Chapter 5, Therapy).

Nonpustular psoriasis: localized
29–37 Legs and knees.

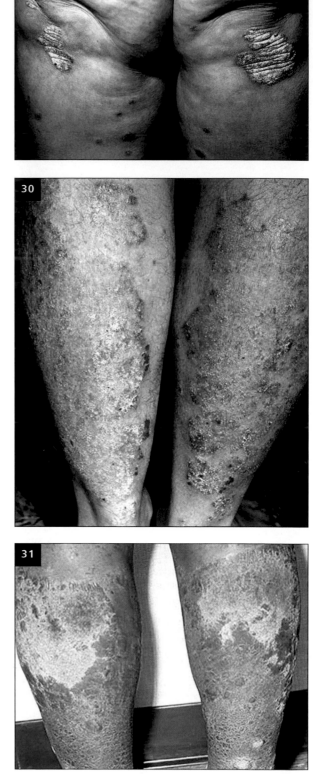

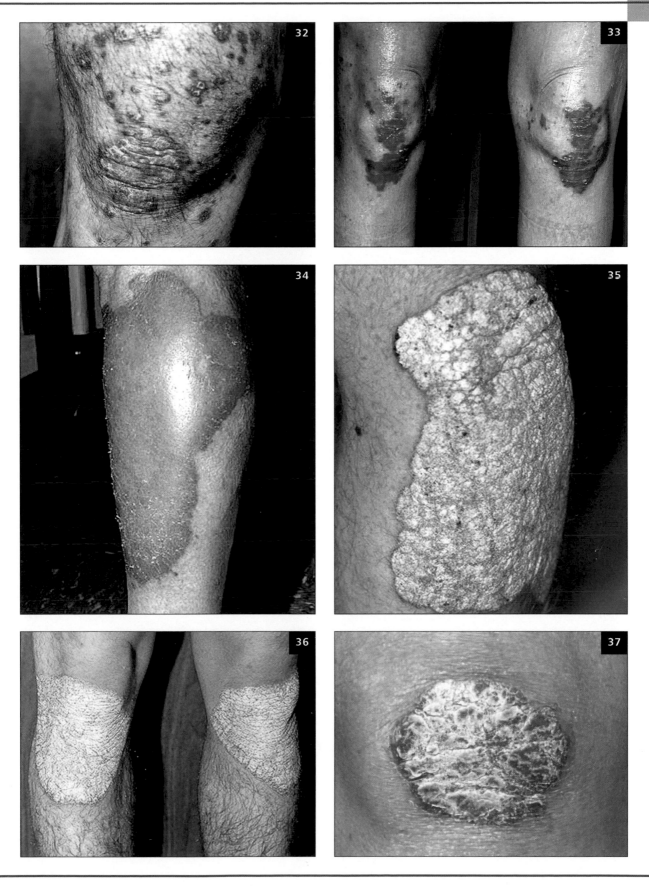

Nonpustular psoriasis: localized

38–45 Arms and elbows.
46–48 Umbilicus.

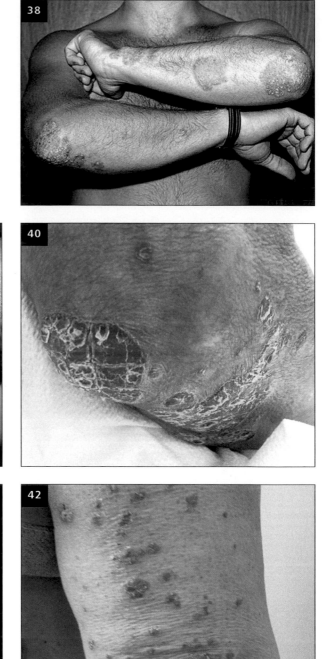

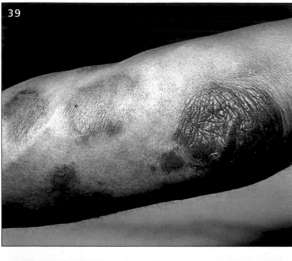

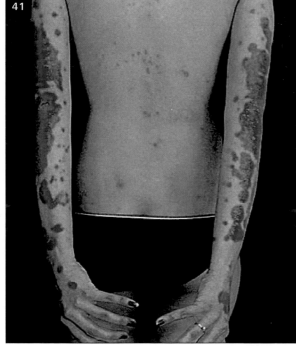

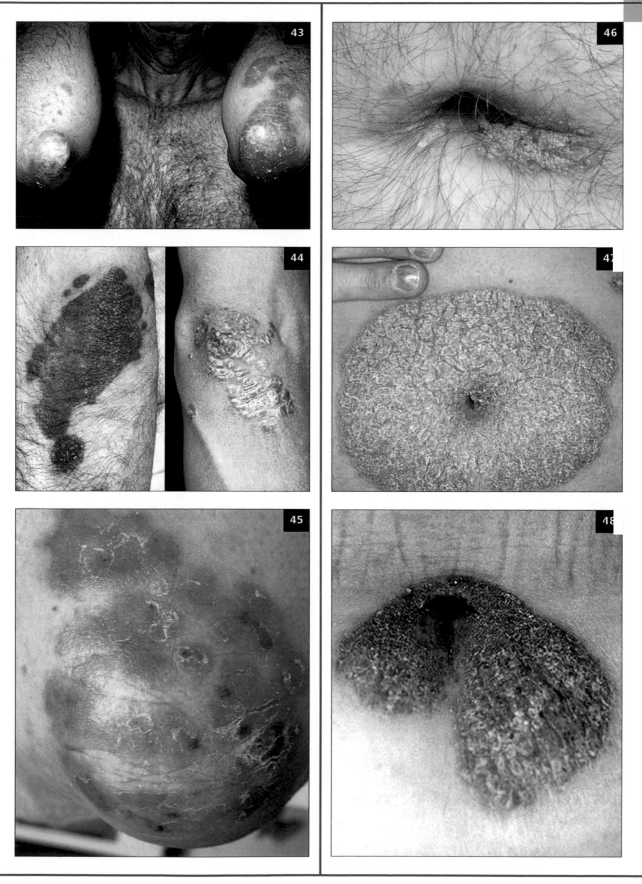

Nonpustular psoriasis: localized
49, 50 Buttocks.
51–59 Face.

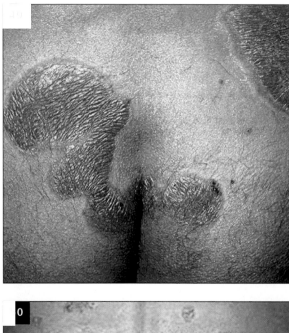

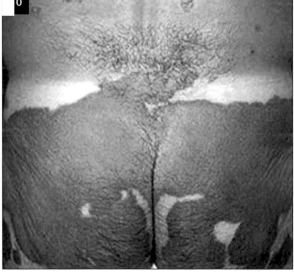

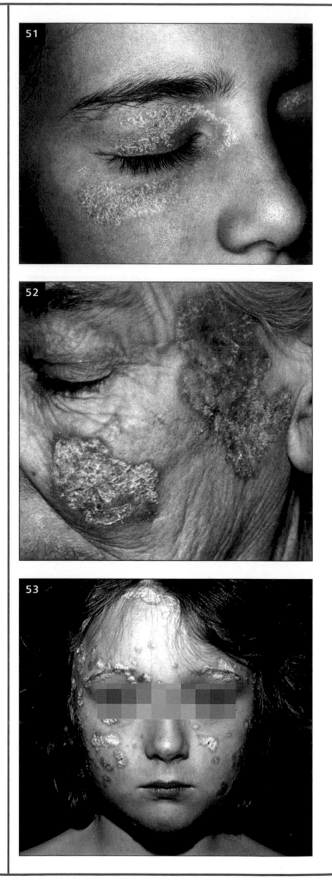

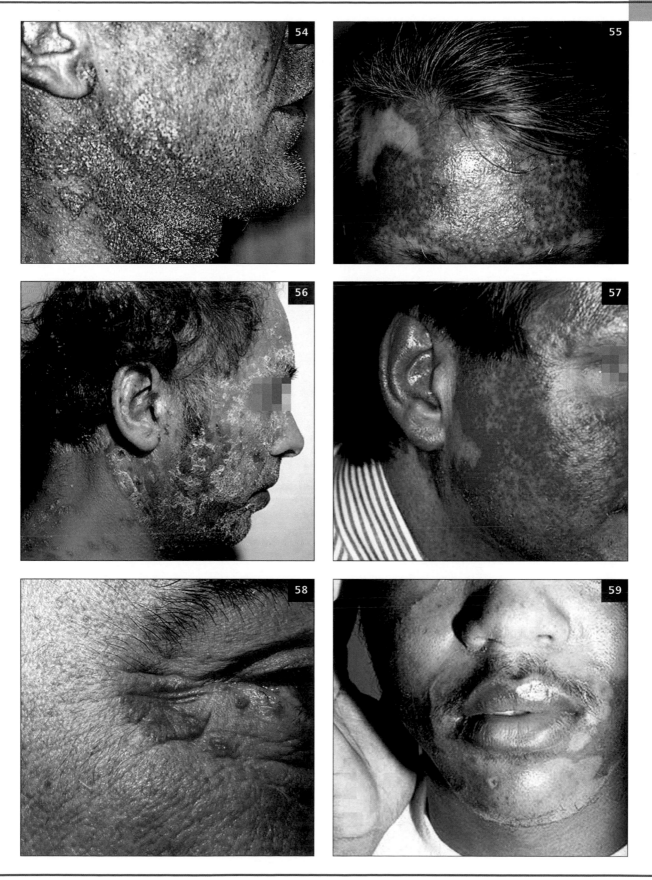

Nonpustular psoriasis: localized

60 Neck.

61–64 Tongue. Note the serpiginous borders, which often migrate, leading to the designation 'geographic tongue.'

65–70 Ears. Lesions favor the conchal bowl and posterior auricular area,

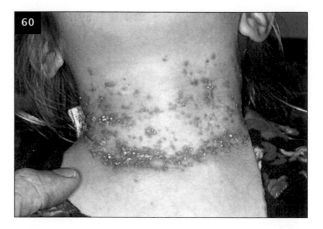

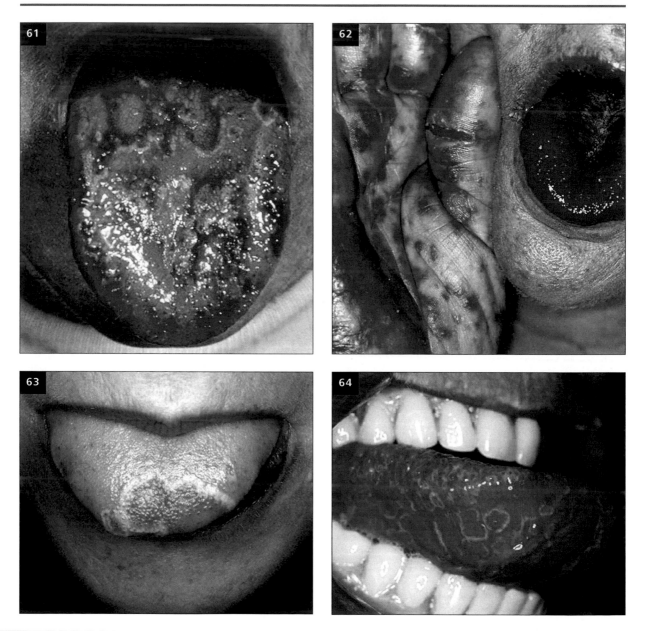

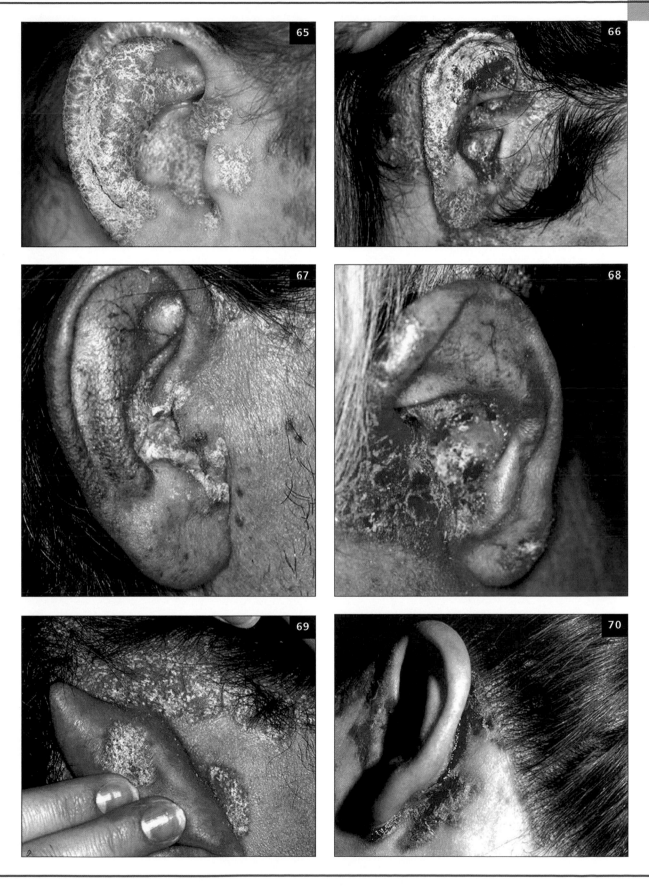

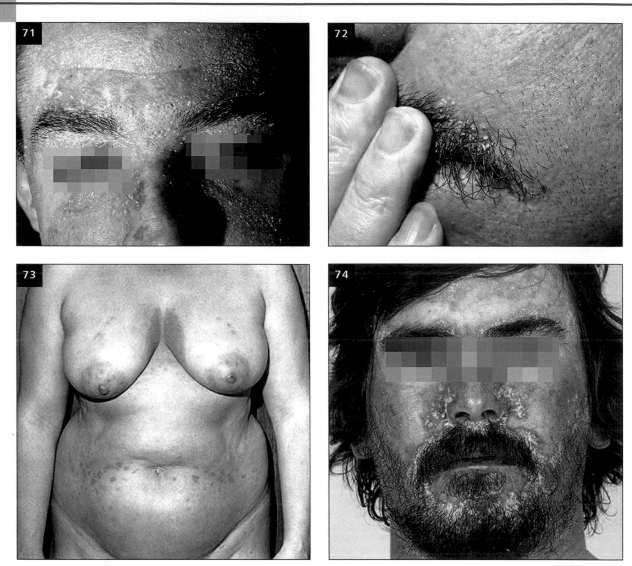

Nonpustular psoriasis: localized

71–74 Sebo-psoriasis. This subtype resembles seborrheic dermatitis.

75–80 Flexural distribution.

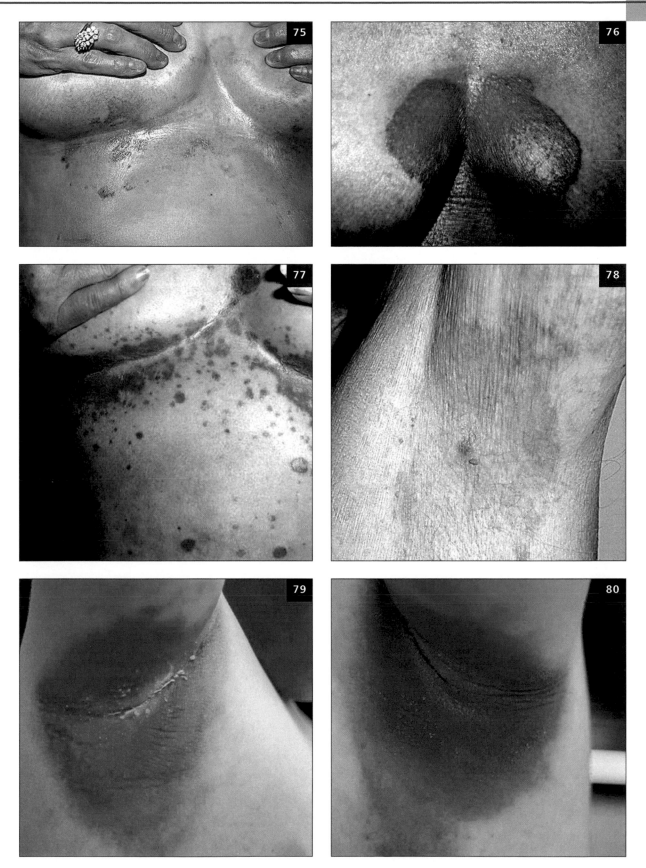

Nonpustular psoriasis: localized

81–86 Flexural and genital distribution.

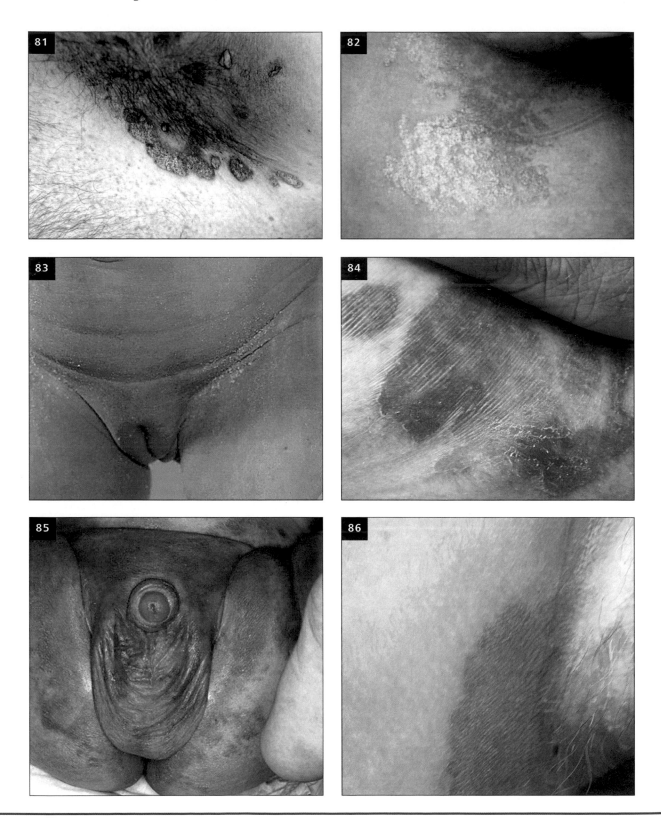

Nonpustular psoriasis: localized

87–92 Scalp psoriasis. Lesions may extend for small distances beyond the hairline.

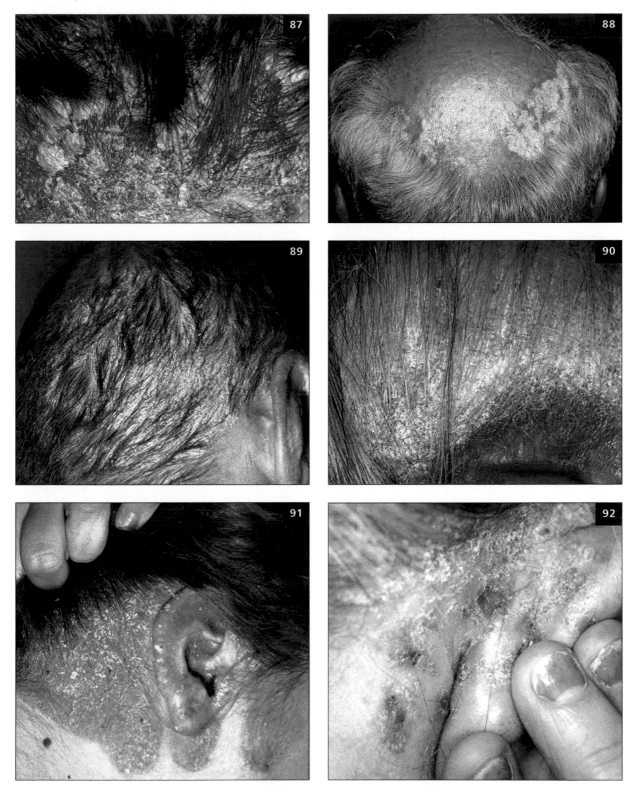

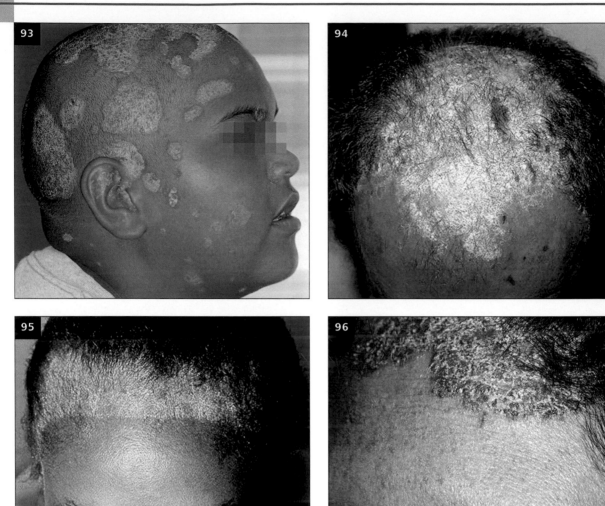

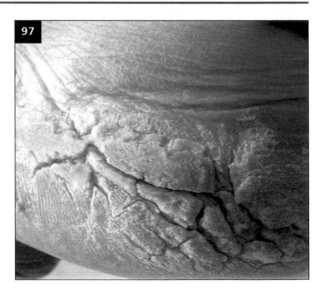

Nonpustular psoriasis: localized

93–96 Scalp psoriasis.

97–102 Nonpustular, hyperkeratotic, palmoplantar psoriasis, involving the feet.

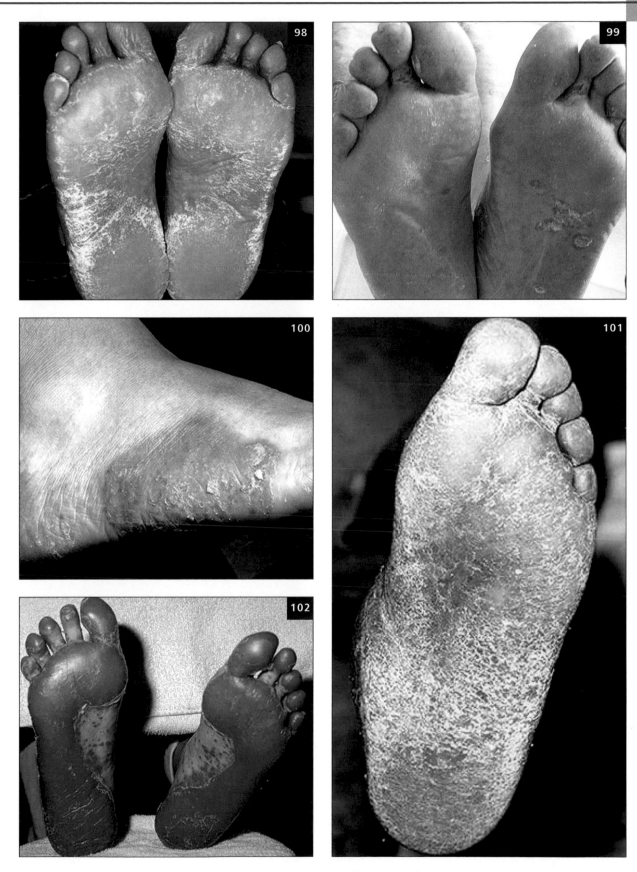

Nonpustular psoriasis: localized

103–108 Nonpustular palmoplantar psoriasis, involving the hands.

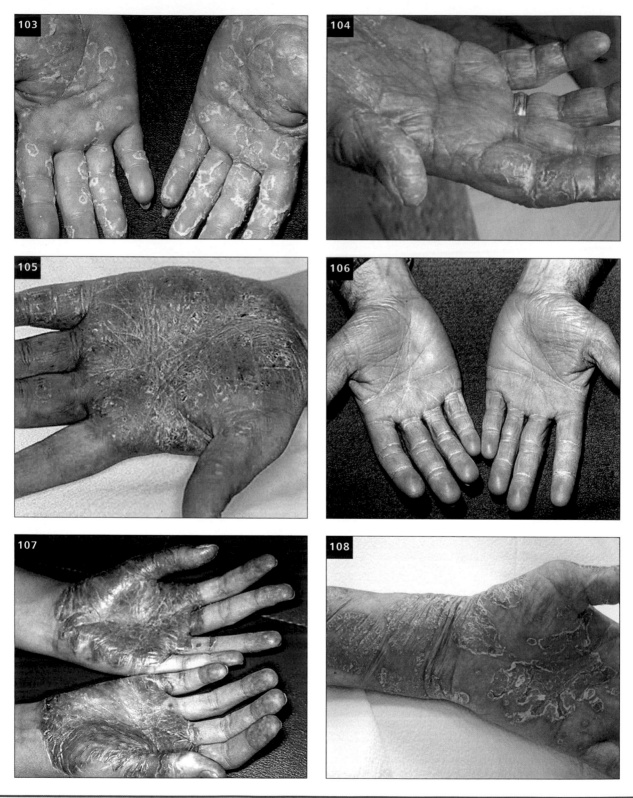

Nonpustular psoriasis: generalized

109–114 Guttate psoriasis.

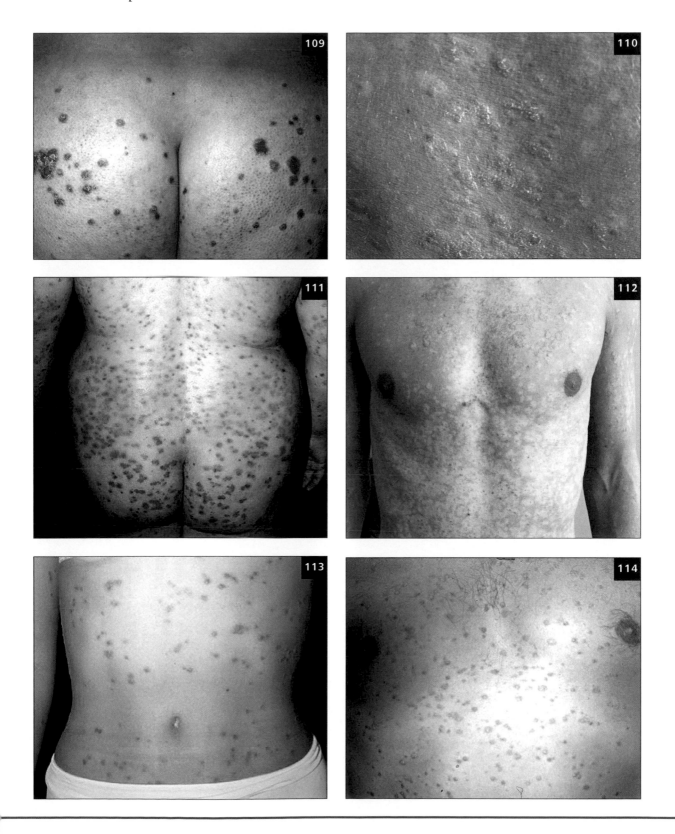

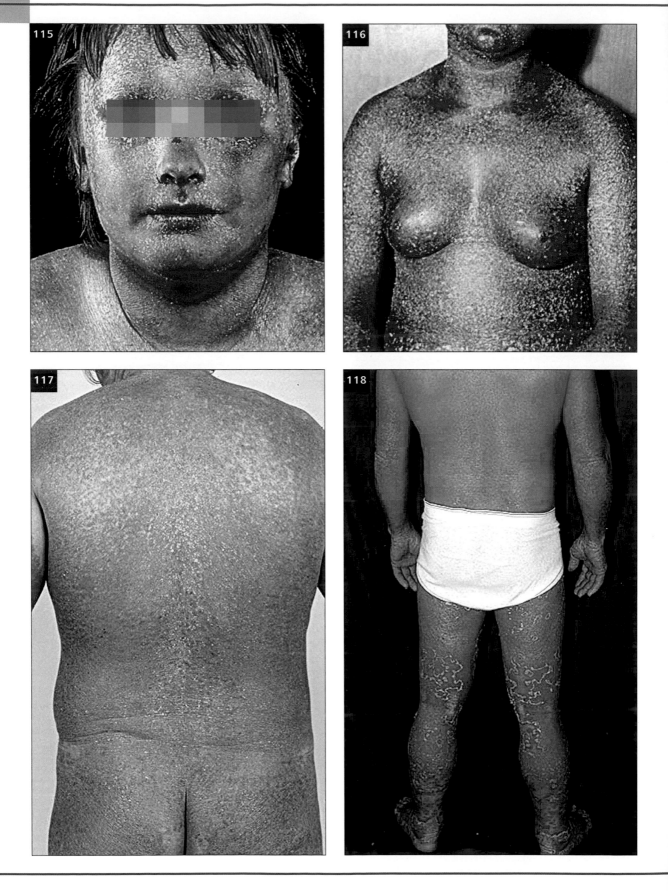

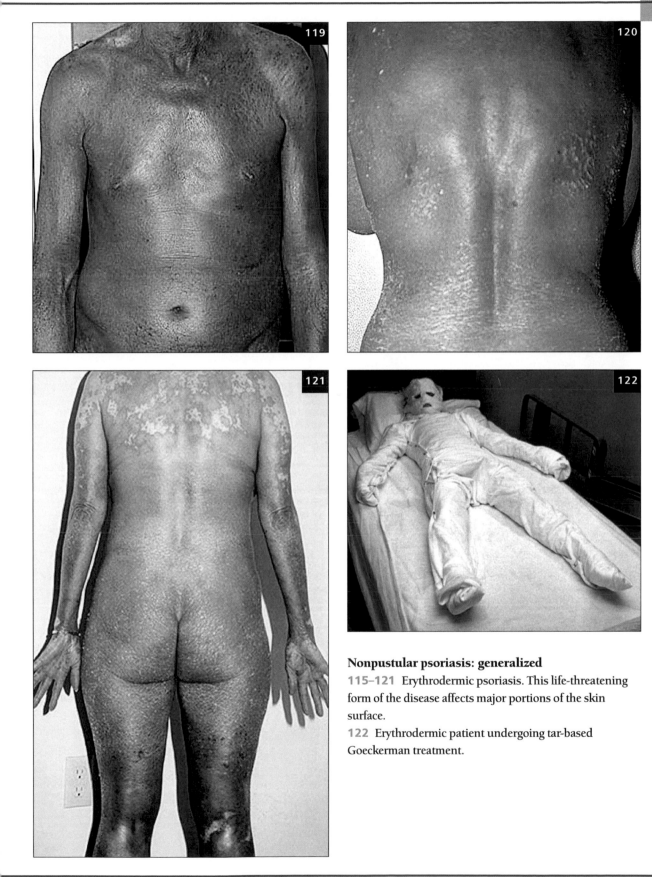

Nonpustular psoriasis: generalized

115–121 Erythrodermic psoriasis. This life-threatening form of the disease affects major portions of the skin surface.

122 Erythrodermic patient undergoing tar-based Goeckerman treatment.

Pustular psoriasis: localized

123–132 Pustular palmoplantar psoriasis; feet.

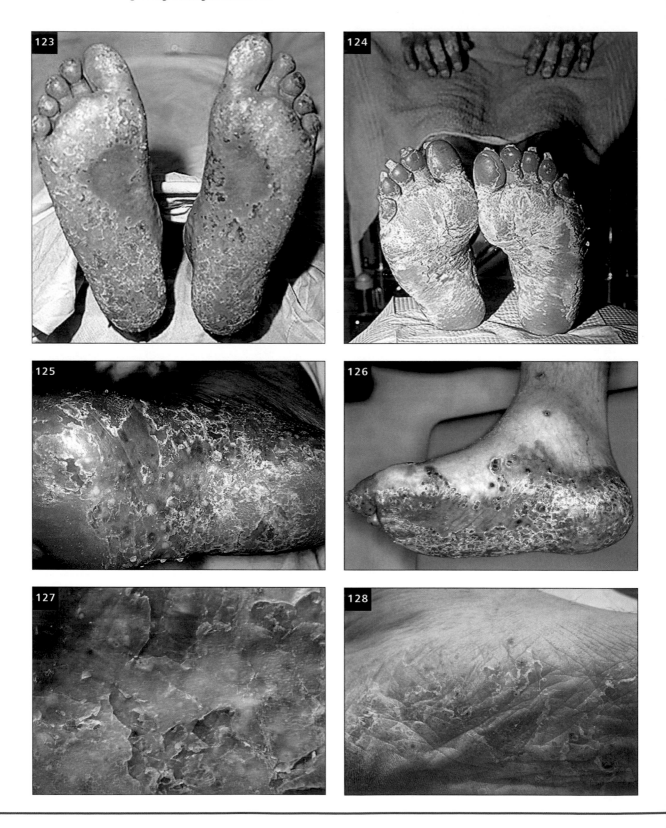

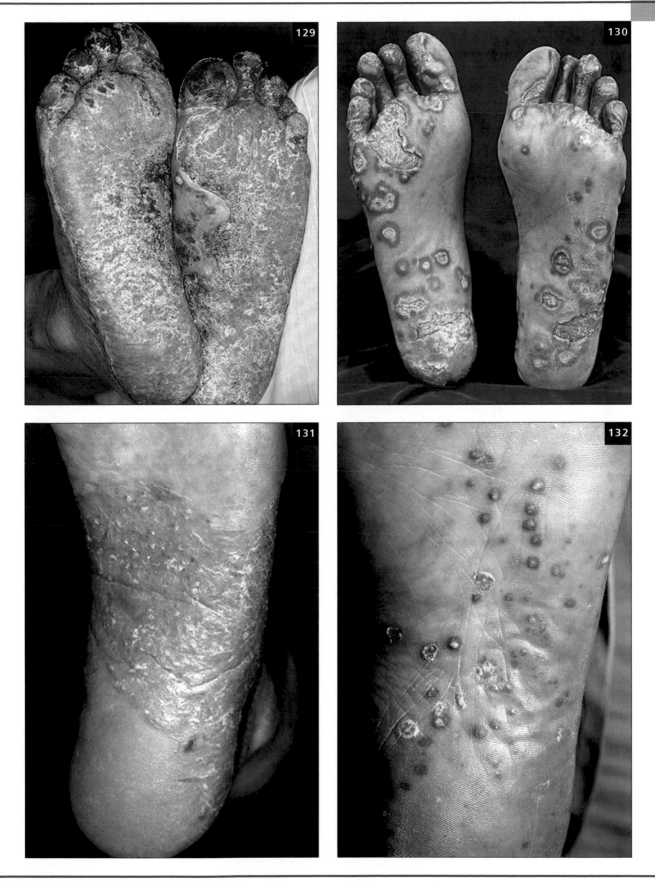

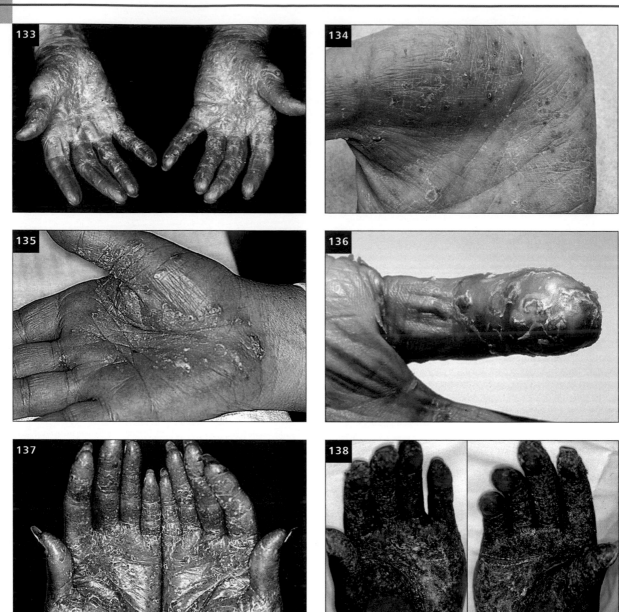

Pustular psoriasis: localized

133–138 Pustular palmoplantar psoriasis; hands.
139–146 Acrodermatitis continua of Hallopeau.

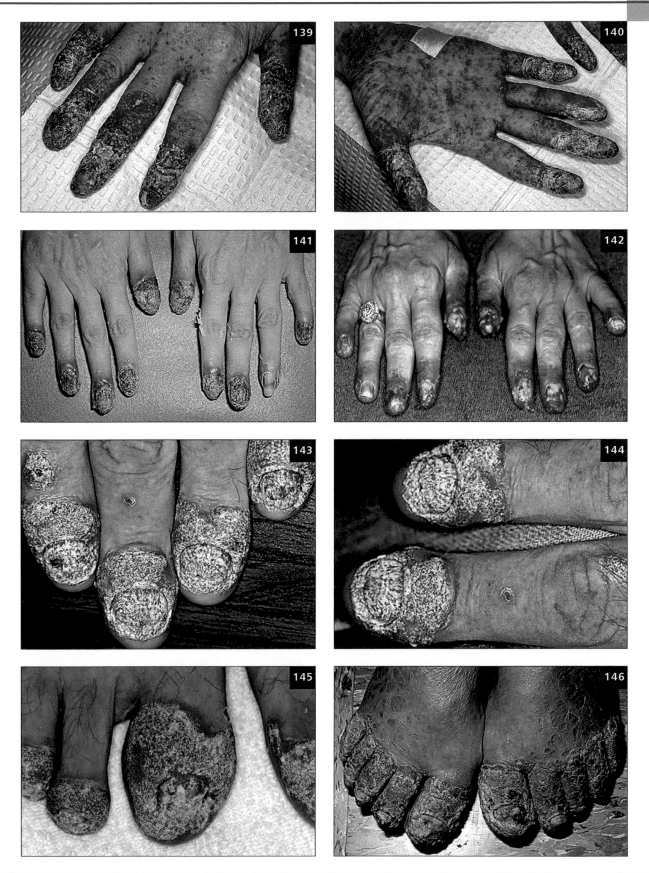

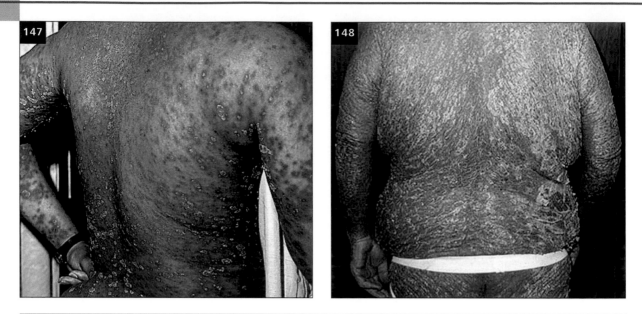

Pustular psoriasis: generalized

147, 148 'von Zumbusch-type' psoriasis.

Other descriptors: nail disease

149–152 Nail pitting.
153–156 Onycholysis.
157, 158 Oil drops.
159–160 Subungual hyperkeratosis.

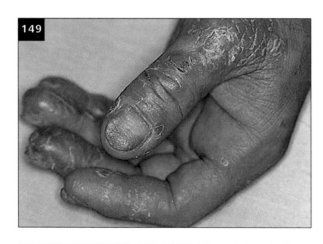

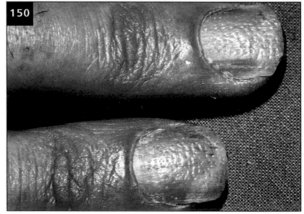

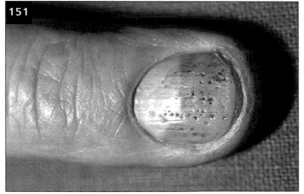

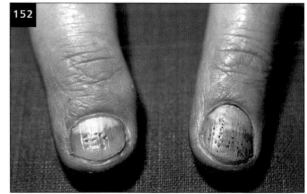

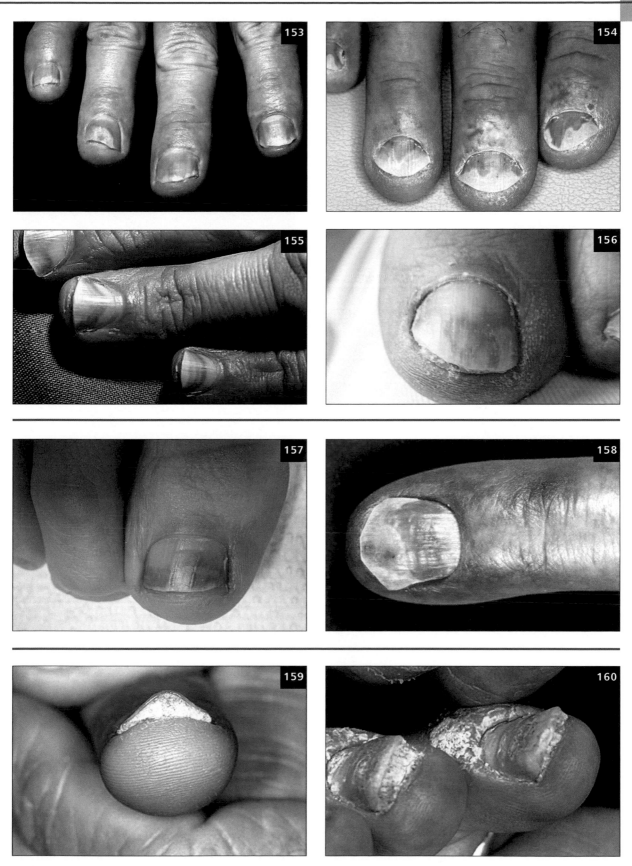

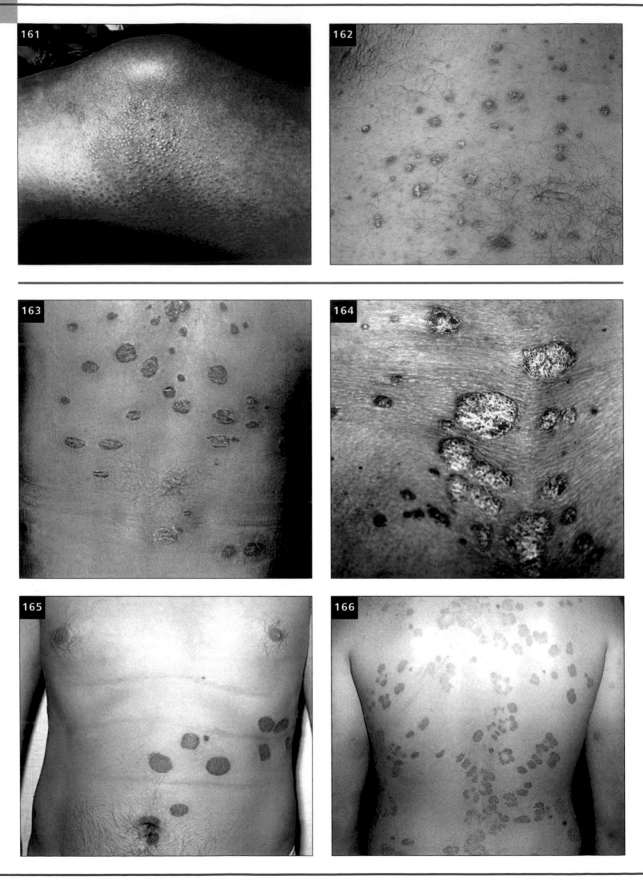

Other descriptors: small versus large plaques

161, 162 Follicular psoriasis.

163–166 Small plaque psoriasis.

167–171 Large plaque psoriasis, with confluence, producing 'geographic' forms.

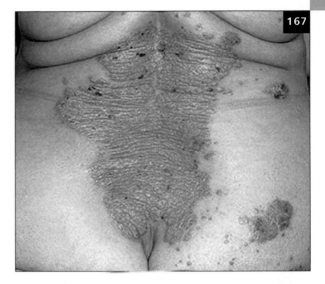

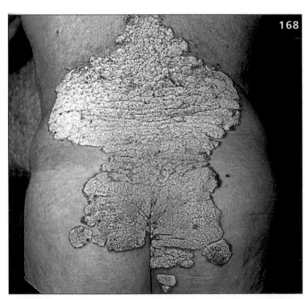

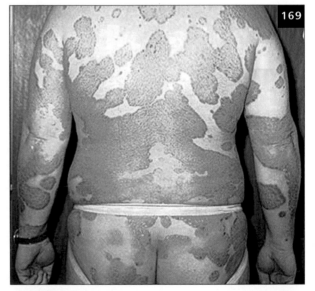

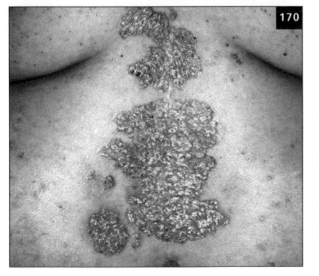

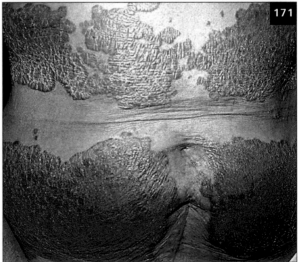

Other descriptors: stable versus unstable disease

172–180 Unstable, inflammatory forms of psoriasis.

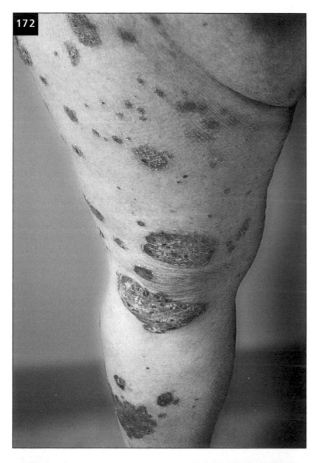

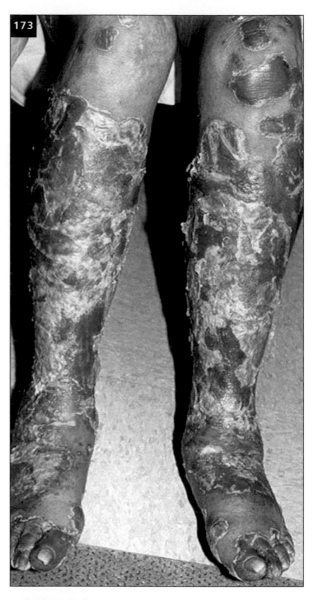

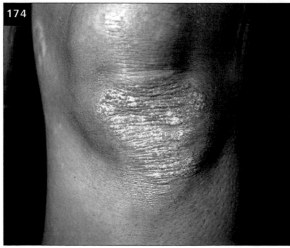

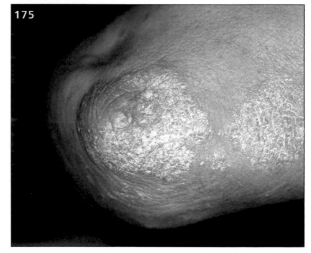

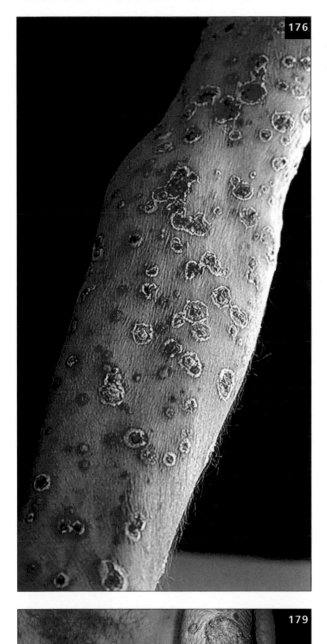

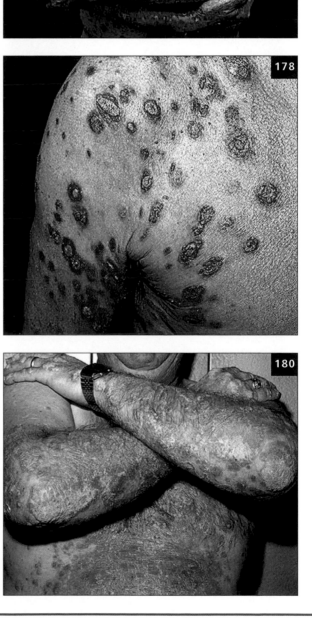

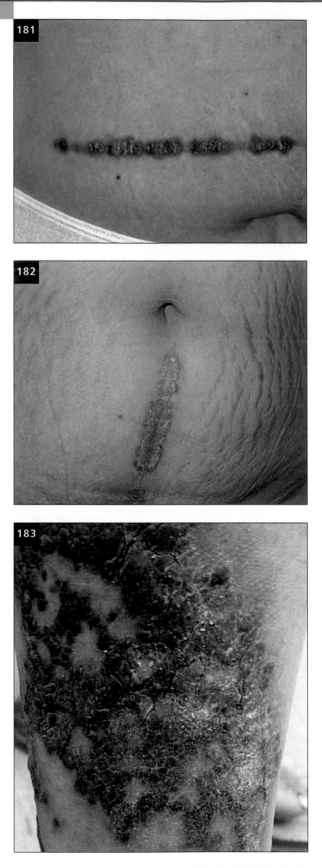

Other descriptors: stable versus unstable disease
181–183 Koebner phenomenon. Psoriasis lesions may develop at sites of injury or scarring.

3 DIFFERENTIAL DIAGNOSIS

STUDENTS OF PSORIASIS have struggled for centuries to distinguish the disease from its 'mimics.' With a wide range of clinical presentations, psoriasis may resemble many other dermatoses, inflammatory, infectious, and neoplastic. Characteristics that hint at the presence of psoriasis include family history, aspects of symmetry, distribution, silvery scaling, and nail changes[1]. Some diseases, however, emulate the appearance of psoriasis so closely that a therapeutic trial of topical therapy may be necessary. If uncertainty persists, biopsy, culture, and selected laboratory tests may aid in confirming the presence or absence of psoriasis. Fortunately, with time, the vast majority of cases of psoriasis declare themselves, evolving into the classic form (*Table 7*).

Table 7 Psoriasis mimickers with differentiating features.

Mimics	Features distinct from psoriasis
INFLAMMATORY	
Atopic dermatitis	Flexural distribution, degree of erythema, 'weeping' lesions, lack of scale and lesser nail disease, significant pruritis, personal and/or family history of atopy
Dyshidrotic eczema	Vesicles with 'tapioca'-like fluid, involvement of sides of fingers, toes and webs, significant pruritus
Nummular eczema	Lesions do not expand, less silvery scale and erythema, uniform size, distal leg a common site
Pityriasis rubra pilaris	Orange hue, follicular orientation, patches of normal skin among diseased skin ('islands of sparing'), less broad array of nail disease (no pitting, onycholysis, or 'oil drop'), hyperkeratotic palms and soles (yellowish)
Pityriasis rosea	Presence of 'herald patch,' 'Christmas tree' distribution, collarette of scale, salmon color, self-limiting 2–3 months' course
INFECTIOUS	
Tinea capitis	Alopecia, broken hair shafts, possible adenopathy
Tinea corporis/tinea cruris	Active scaly border, central clearing, asymmetry
Tinea pedis	Involvement of lateral web space, unilaterality, vesicular, 'moccasin'-type diffuse scaling
Tinea unguium	Asymmetry, predominantly toenails, lack of pitting
Candida	Peripheral pustules ('satellite' pustules), moist, whitish appearance, involvement of crural areas and finger webs
Candida of genitalia ('balanitis')	Pustules, diffuse erythema, erosions and fissures
Secondary syphilis	Early erythematous exanthem, copper-colored lesions ('pennies') on palms and soles, mucosal lesions, condyloma lata, history of chancre
NEOPLASTIC	
Squamous cell carcinoma *in-situ* (Bowen's disease)	Sun-exposed distribution, lesions few in number, gradual increase in size, resistant to treatment, potential progression to erosions
Cutaneous T-cell lymphoma (CTCL)	Often initially diagnosed as psoriasis; asymmetry, more irregular and fewer lesions, wrinkled appearance, 'bathing-trunk' distribution common, unresponsive to traditional topical therapies, potential progression to plaques, nodules and tumors

INFLAMMATORY SKIN DISEASE

Eczema

Eczema appears at the top of the list of dermatoses causing confusion with psoriasis. Although many forms exist, three types – atopic, dyshidrotic, and nummular – particularly resemble subtypes of psoriasis.

Atopic dermatitis

A multifactorial condition beginning in childhood, atopic dermatitis (AD) manifests in a variety of ways depending on age and severity. In children under 2 years, characteristic plaques with vibrant erythema and minor scale appear on the face and extensor surfaces of the limbs. In older patients, distribution becomes flexural and plaques thickened with exaggerated skin markings (lichenification), the result of chronic excoriation. Patients report a long personal and/or family history of asthma and allergic rhinitis, known as the atopic diathesis. Paramount among the subjective aspects of the disease, pruritus may be triggered by changes in temperature or humidity. Contact with irritants, such as water, or allergens may also exacerbate symptoms. Indeed, pruritus with resultant excoriation often incites characteristic lesions, leading to the lay description of atopic dermatitis as 'the itch that rashes.' Beyond flexural surfaces, other sites of involvement include periorbital and perioral areas, as well as the hands. Nails may be affected, although typically to a mild degree. Despite similarities with psoriasis, AD remains distinct. Key differentiating features of AD include characteristic history, severe pruritus, distribution of lesions, marked erythema, as well as paucity of scale and nail changes[2–4]. Often lesions are 'weepy' or secondarily infected (impetiginized). Topical steroids

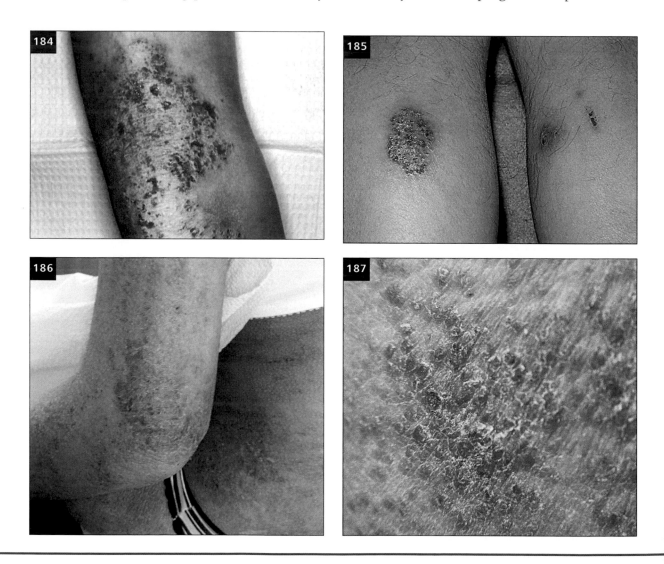

and emollients are mainstays of treatment with topical immunomodulating agents and systemic antipruritics important additions. In severe cases, systemic corticosteroids, cyclosporin or, on occasion, even azathioprine and mycophenolate mofetil are utilized (**184–191**)[5].

Dyshidrotic eczema

Dyshidrotic eczema, also known as pompholyx, causes symmetric, bilateral vesiculation of the hands and feet. One of the few lesions resembling palmoplantar pustular psoriasis, dyshidrotic vesicles evolve into punctate, scaly papules and even pustules[5]. The 'tapioca-like' vesicular fluid, intense pruritus, and involvement of the finger webs and dorsal hands differentiate dyshidrosis from its psoriatic counterpart. Morbidity is great and treatment difficult (**192–196**).

Nummular eczema

A puzzling relative of atopic dermatitis, nummular eczema presents with disk-shaped, scaly plaques frequently on the extremities. Unlike psoriatic plaques, lesions of nummular eczema typically do not expand[1]. Scale is also less exuberant and erythema less uniform. Like AD, nummular eczema may cause extreme pruritus, especially in the elderly (**197–200**).

Eczema versus psoriasis
184–187 Atopic dermatitis. Compared with psoriasis, lesions tend to be less vivid, well-defined, and scaly.
188–191 Psoriasis.

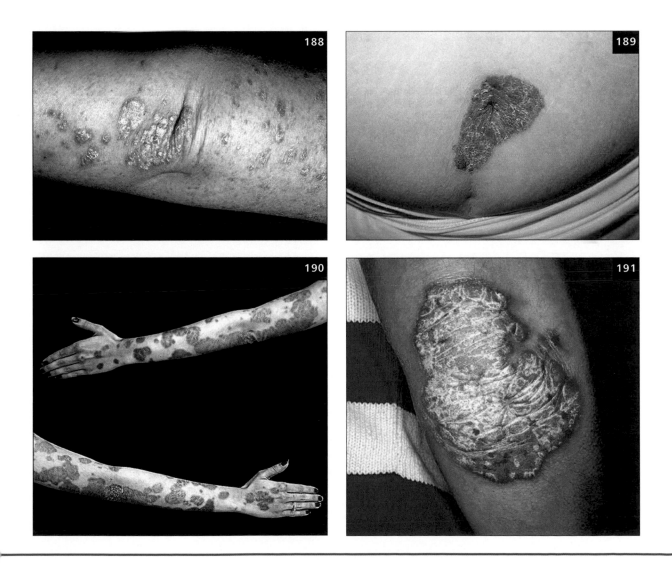

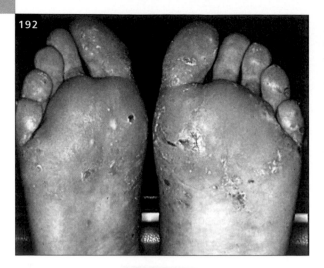

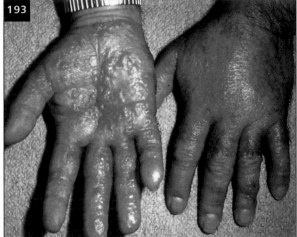

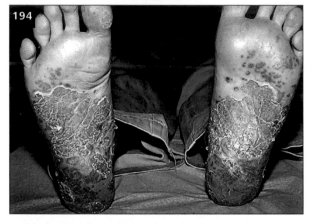

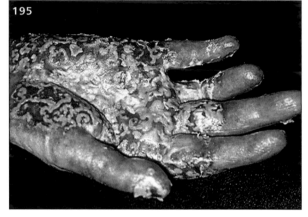

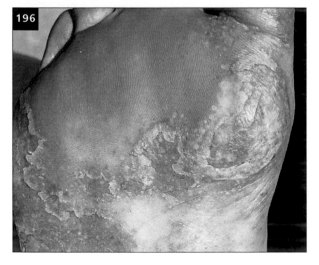

Pityriasis rosea

A self-limited, inflammatory disease possibly related to infection with human herpes virus 6 and 7, pityriasis rosea (PR) begins with a 2–10-cm, salmon-red plaque usually on the trunk, known as the 'herald patch.' The plaque precedes the eruption of smaller (1–2-cm) patches, papules, and thin plaques on the trunk and proximal extremities, developing 1–2 weeks later. Classically, lesions develop along skin cleavage lines and display a thin rim of scale. This 'Christmas-tree' distribution and 'collarette' of scale help to distinguish PR from guttate psoriasis. The eruption is usually self-limited, lasting 2–3 months (**201, 202**).

Eczema versus psoriasis

192, 193 Dyshidrotic eczema. Note the characteristic clear vesicles.

194–196 Palmoplantar pustular psoriasis with yellowish pustules.

Eczema versus psoriasis

197 Nummular eczema. Lesions are thin, moist, and lack silvery scale.

198–200 Small-plaque psoriasis.

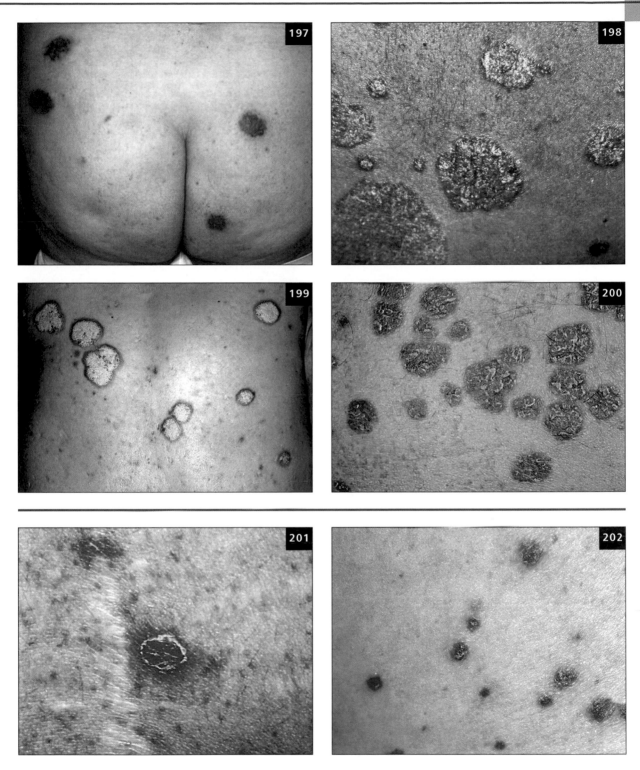

Pityriasis rosea versus psoriasis

201 Pityriasis rosea. The peripheral rim of scale is a distinguishing feature.

202 Guttate psoriasis. Gentle scraping of the surface will elicit silvery scale.

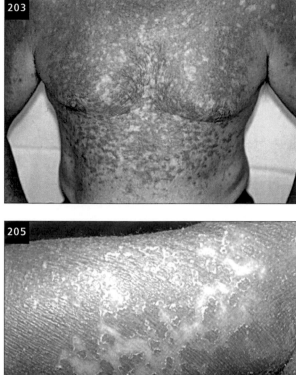

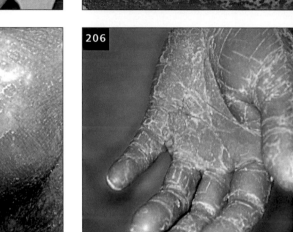

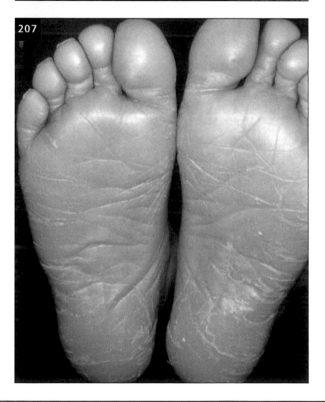

Pityriasis rubra pilaris versus psoriasis
203–209 Pityriasis rubra pilaris. Note the more yellow-orange hue and follicular appearance.
210–213 Psoriasis.

Pityriasis rubra pilaris

The scaly plaques of pityriasis rubra pilaris (PRP) strongly evoke psoriasis. Indeed, PRP was originally described as a psoriasis subtype[6]. Decades later, dermatologists began to appreciate the distinct orange hue and follicular distribution of PRP. Waxy plaques affect the palms, soles, trunk, limbs, and scalp. Despite often extensive disease, patches of normal skin intermingle, known as 'islands of sparing.' Nails may demonstrate subungual debris, as with psoriasis, but lack pitting, oil drops, and onycholysis[7]. In sum, distinguishing features of PRP include the follicular orientation and color of lesions, 'islands of sparing,' more acral distribution, and narrow range of nail changes. Additionally, PRP may be even more refractory to therapy than psoriasis (203–213).

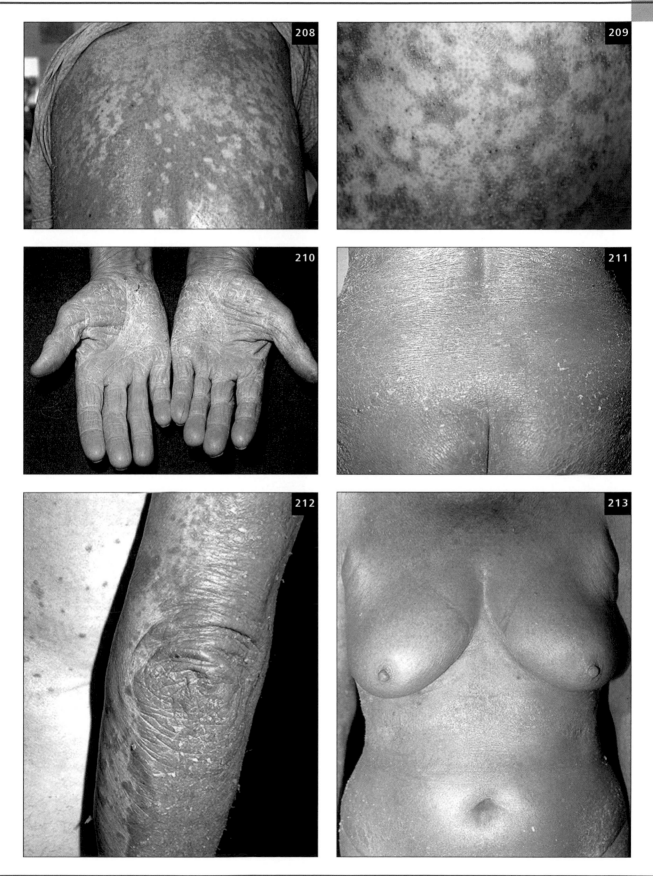

INFECTIOUS DISORDERS

Dermatophye infection

A diverse group of fungi, the dermatophytes, also termed 'tinea,' infect keratinized tissues of the skin, hair, and nails. While the clinical manifestations of dermatophytic infection range widely, many features mimic psoriasis. Infection of the skin and hair can lead to erythematous, scaly plaques with an active border, typical of psoriasis. Nail involvement may present with subungual hyperkeratosis identical to psoriatic nail disease. The astute clinician, however, will note asymmetry of dermatophytic lesions, as well as subtle differences in the quality of the active border and central clearing.

Tinea capitis

A disease mainly of young children, tinea capitis evolves from infection of the scalp hair shaft by a dermatophyte, most commonly *Trichophyton tonsurans*[8]. Of the various manifestations of tinea capitis, the noninflammatory subtypes are most often confused with psoriasis. Lesions appear circular with abundant scale and relatively sharp demarcation. Alopecia with broken hair shafts also hints at tinea. Regional lymphadenopathy may be present with more inflammatory forms. Wood's lamp examination and microscopy of affected hairs is usually sufficient to clinch the diagnosis, with fungal cultures occasionally required. Oral, not topical, antifungals are the standard treatment (**214–217**).

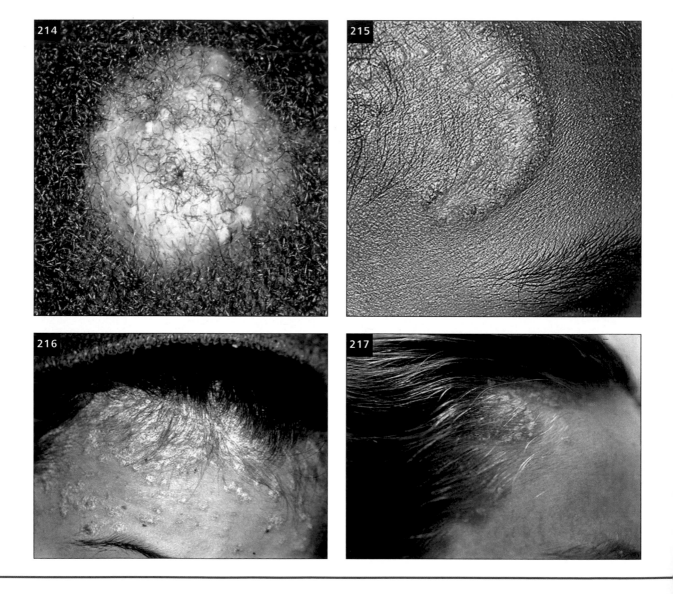

Tinea corporis

Dermatophytoses of the skin subdivide according to anatomic location, with separate designations for the groin, feet, hands, and all other surfaces. Tinea corporis, for instance, refers to dermatophyte infection of any epidermal location other than the scalp, groin, feet, or hands. *Trichophyton rubrum* is the most common culprit[8]. Circular or annular asymmetric plaques produce marked erythema and scale. As with other dermatophytoses, the border appears relatively more 'active' than the remainder of the lesion. Microscopic evaluation with the application of potassium hydroxide (KOH) to a collection of scale collected from the active border followed by gentle heating will reveal septate hyphae. Biopsy specimen treated with periodic-acid Schiff (PAS) may be more sensitive for the detection of fungi[8]. Unlike hair and nail dermatophytosis, treatment with topical antifungals is normally adequate (**218, 219**).

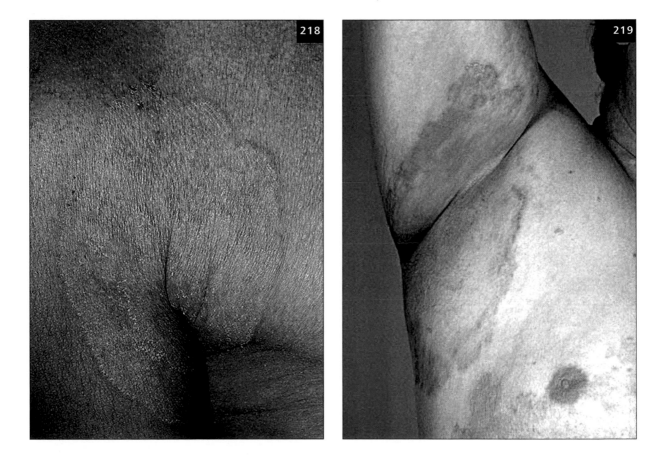

Dermatophyte infection versus psoriasis

214, 215 Tinea capitis. Alopecia and minor scaling are clues to diagnosis

216, 217 Scalp psoriasis.

218 Tinea corporis. Note the active, scaly border.

219 Flexural psoriasis; minimal scale noted in this form.

Tinea cruris

Closely related tinea cruris differs from the corporal subtype in anatomic location (groin), relative paucity of scale except at the border, and propensity for confluence of plaques. As with tinea corporis, *T. rubrum* causes most cases[8]. The diagnostic approach and treatment options are similar (**220–222**).

Tinea pedis

Excessive moisture predisposes to dermatophyte infection of the foot, known as tinea pedis or 'athlete's foot.' Several categories exist, however, the so-called 'moccasin-type' most closely resembles nonpustular, plantar psoriasis. Fine, whitish scale and leathery hyperkeratosis encasing the foot characterize the clinical appearance of this type of tinea pedis. Other manifestations of dermatophytosis may coexist, such as interdigital and bullous lesions, which distinguish the infection from psoriasis (**223–226**).

Tinea unguium

Tinea unguium refers to dermatophyte infection of the nail, also termed 'onychomycosis.' In its primary form, tinea unguium affects healthy nails causing discoloration and subungual hyperkeratosis similar to psoriatic nail disease. Alternatively, pre-existing nail damage, such as onycholysis in psoriatics, predisposes to secondary onychomycosis, leading the two conditions to often coexist. Patients with depressed immunity, such as those with diabetes and HIV/AIDS, are prone to infection, usually by *T. rubrum* or *T. mentagrophytes*[8]. While often indistinguishable from nail psoriasis, tinea unguium may be differentiated by asymmetry, sparing of the fingernails, and lack of pitting. A KOH preparation of clippings from the nail bed may secure the diagnosis, but PAS staining of clippings and/or fungal culture of debris are often required (**227–230**).

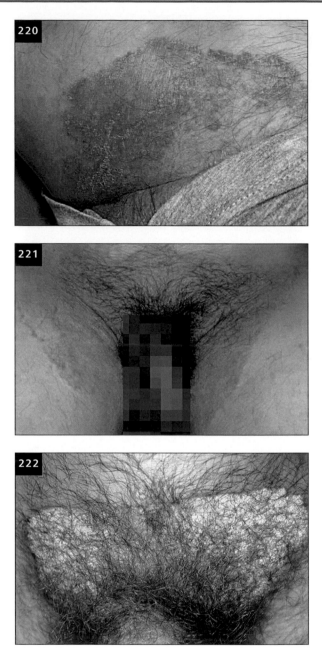

Dermatophyte infection versus psoriasis
220 Tinea cruris in a psoriasis patient using topical corticosteroids.
221 Tinea cruris. The relative paucity of scale differentiates this from psoriasis.
222 Psoriasis of the groin.
223, 224 Tinea pedis. Note the asymmetry and web involvement.
225, 226 Psoriasis of the foot.
227, 228 Tinea unguium. Pitting is not observed.
229, 230 Nail psoriasis.

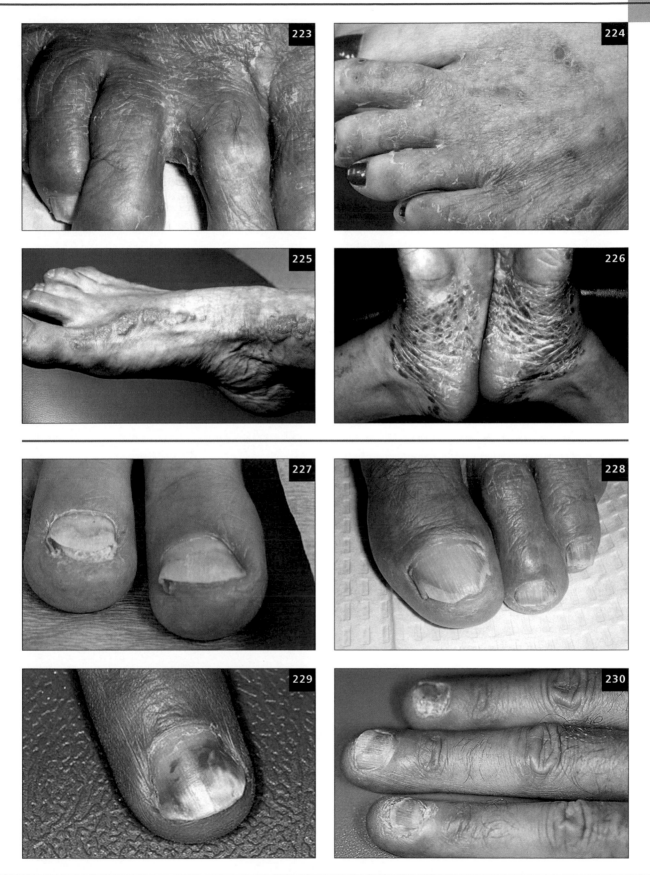

Candida infection

Another infectious psoriasis mimic, the yeast species *Candida albicans* affects warm, moist areas of the body, including axillae, inguinal folds, gluteal cleft, perineum, finger webs, angles of the mouth, and breast folds. Erythematous papules coalesce to form eroded plaques with characteristic peripheral pustules. These so-called 'satellite' pustules distinguish cutaneous candidiasis from psoriasis. A KOH preparation reveals budding yeast with 'pseudohyphae,' confirming the diagnosis. Keeping affected areas dry and use of topical anti-candidal agents are first-line treatments (**231–237**).

Candida also affects the nonkeratinized epithelium of the genitals, as does psoriasis. The term 'balanitis' refers to candidiasis of the prepuce and glans penis. Discrete or coalescent pustules develop on erythematous, often eroded, skin. Diffuse erythema and pustules suggest balanitis as opposed to psoriasis. Diagnosis is often made clinically (**238, 239**).

Secondary syphilis

With its multitude of expressions involving the skin and other organ systems, syphilis is known as 'the great imitator.' Secondary syphilis, developing in untreated patients 2–6 months after initial infection with the spirochete, may very closely resemble guttate psoriasis and pityriasis rosea. Interestingly, patients with early secondary syphilis develop a faint, erythematous exanthema prior to the guttate-like papular eruption. In the latter, copper-colored papules of various sizes up to 1 cm develop gradually over the trunk and limbs, ultimately involving the palms and soles. Lesions characteristically lack signs of inflammation, but scaling may be present. Mucosal lesions, especially on the mouth and genitalia, are frequent. A typical eruption in the setting of a positive screening, followed by treponemal antibody test confirms the diagnosis. Though rarely performed, dark field microscopy of samples from papular lesions will demonstrate spirochetes (**240, 241**).

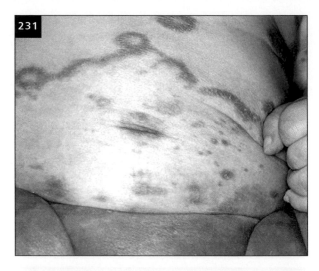

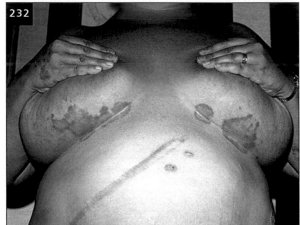

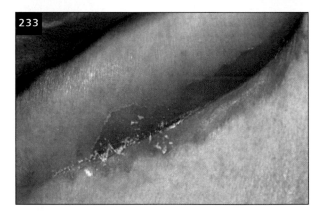

Candida infection versus psoriasis
231–233 Psoriasis.
234–237 Candidiasis. Note the discrete pustules at the periphery.
238 Balanitis. Note the moist, non-scaly quality of the lesion.
239 Psoriasis of the genitals.

Secondary syphilis versus psoriasis
240 Secondary syphilis. The characteristic copper color of the lesions distinguishes the eruption from psoriasis. Palms and soles are frequently involved.
241 Guttate psoriasis.

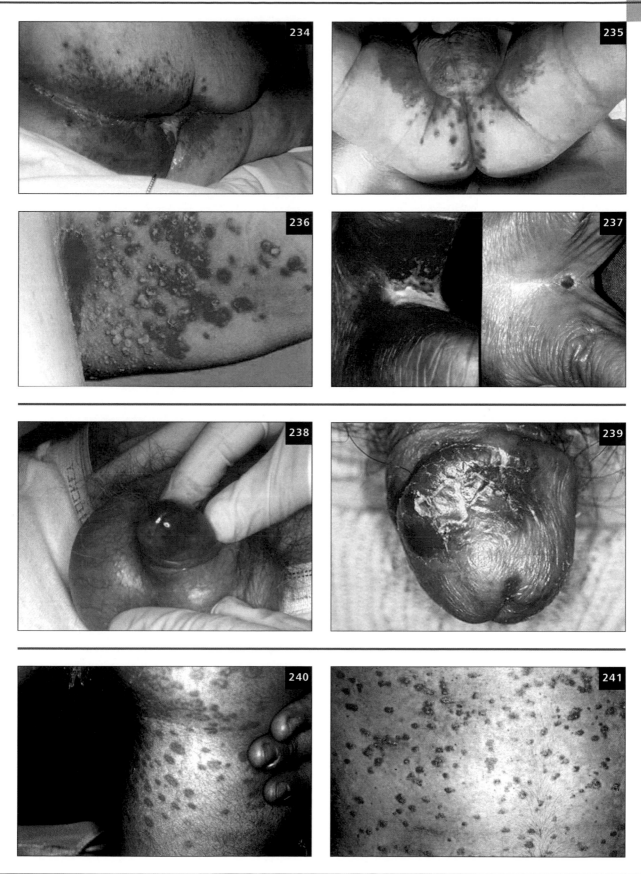

NEOPLASMS

Most ominous of the masquerade syndromes, neoplasms affecting the skin may cause scaly, erythematous plaques identical to psoriasis. Lesions may be so similar, in fact, that only resistance to treatment guides the clinician away from a diagnosis of chronic psoriasis and toward consideration of neoplasia. In such cases, histology aids in the diagnosis, although sequential biopsies may be required (see below).

Squamous cell carcinoma *in situ*

Well-circumscribed, isolated erythematous plaques with scale just as adequately describes the lesions of squamous cell carcinoma *in situ* (SCCIS), or Bowen's disease, as psoriasis. Lesions favor areas of sun damage, a risk factor for Bowen's disease, including the ears, scalp, lower lip, upper chest, back, and hands. Males appear more likely to develop SCCIS on the head and neck, whereas women the lower extremities[9]. Other exposures increasing risk include human papilloma virus (HPV), arsenic, heating devices, and iatrogenic radiation. Treatment recalcitrance and/or progression to invasive disease suggest Bowen's disease rather than psoriasis. Paucity of scale, which is less than silvery, as well as a dull background of erythema aid in distinguishing SCCIS from psoriasis (242–244).

Cutaneous T-cell lymphoma

A rare neoplasm of helper T cells, cutaneous T-cell lymphoma (CTCL) encompasses a variety of related conditions, including mycosis fungoides, lymphoma cutis, and Sézary syndrome. Erythematous patches may progress to plaques, which may slowly evolve into nodules or tumors and, in some cases, erythroderma. In this final stage, extensive hematological and even visceral involvement may be seen. The early, 'patch' stage of CTCL demonstrates erythematous plaques with mild scale similar to psoriasis or dermatophytoses, hence the term 'mycosis.' Indeed, patients with 'patch' stage CTCL often carry the diagnosis of psoriasis for many years. Further confusing the picture, these lesions may respond well to both topical corticosteroids and phototherapy initially, as with psoriasis. Biopsy specimens during the patch stage may not consistently demonstrate the characteristic epidermotropism (homing of T cells to the epidermis) and activated CD4+ lymphocytes. Consequently, serial biopsies with special studies,

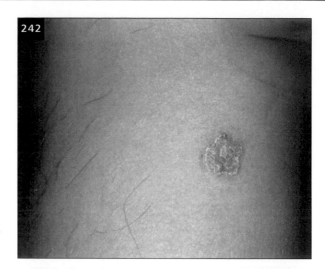

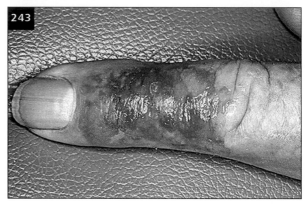

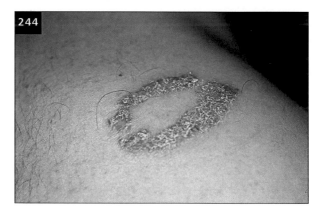

Squamous cell carcinoma versus psoriasis
242, 243 Bowen's disease. Lesions are isolated, well-circumscribed, eroded, and resistant to anti-psoriatic therapies.
244 Annular psoriasis.

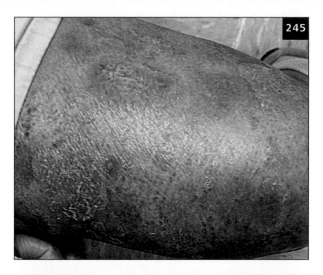

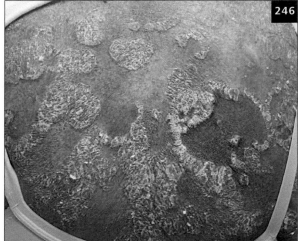

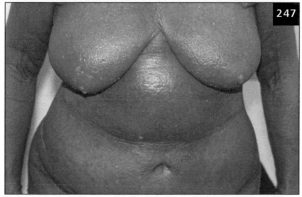

Cutaneous T-cell lymphoma (CTCL) versus psoriasis

245 CTCL; patch stage.
246 CTCL; plaque stage.
247 CTCL; erythroderma.
248, 249 Psoriasis.

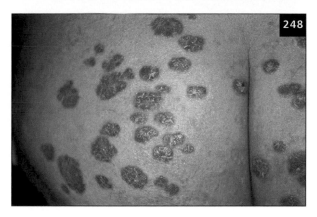

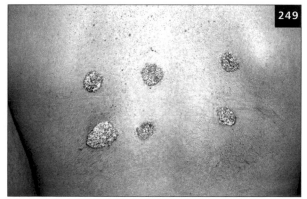

such as T-cell receptor gene rearrangement and flow cytometry, are important for diagnosis.

Thus, the clinician must be wary of the isolated, psoriasiform plaque minimally responsive to topical therapy. If such a lesion raises suspicion for CTCL, initial work-up should include at minimum a full lymph node examination, biopsy of the lesion for routine histology and special studies mentioned above, and complete blood count with peripheral smear. Early lesions respond well to phototherapy, particularly psoralen with ultraviolet A (PUVA). Progression to Sézary syndrome, with generalized erythroderma, warrants consultation with a hematologist/oncologist for appropriate systemic therapy (**245–249**).

4 PSORIATIC ARTHRITIS

Like its cutaneous counterpart, psoriatic arthritis (PsA) has a broad range of clinical manifestations, complex pathophysiology, and deep impact on the quality of life of those afflicted. PsA provides a source of great scientific deliberation and clinical need. Recent advances in epidemiology, immunogenetics, and clinical classification have enhanced our understanding of this enigmatic and often debilitating joint disease.

Discussions of treatment and quality of life considerations related to PsA can be found in the relevant chapters of this book and are not discussed here.

GENERAL DESCRIPTION

PsA joins a unique group of arthritic diseases unified by involvement of the joints and connective tissues of the spine (i.e. spondyloarthropathy), as well as, in most cases, a negative serum test for the rheumatoid factor (RF) antibody to the constant portion of gamma immunoglobulin. A positive test for RF is one of the hallmarks of perhaps the best known of all inflammatory joint diseases, rheumatoid arthritis (RA). Clinicians should be aware, however, that 10–13% of patients with PsA are seropositive for RF[1]. Along with PsA, the so-called 'seronegative spondyloarthropathies' include ankylosing spondylitis, reactive arthritis (Reiter syndrome) and arthritis related to inflammatory bowel disease. Diseases of this group commonly produce signs and symptoms beyond the joints, such as lesions in the mucous membranes, inflammation of the iris and anterior chamber of the eye (i.e. uveitis), aneurysm of aortic root, subclinical inflammatory bowel disease, and diarrhea[2-4].

Despite its inclusion among the seronegative spondyloarthopathies, PsA is unique. Experts in the field suggest that the spine is involved in only a minority of patients with PsA[2] and, when it is, characteristics of symmetry, pain, and movement restriction differentiate the disease from the other spondyloarthropathies (see below). Indeed, many patients with PsA remain free of spinal inflammation altogether and can display a pattern of peripheral joint involvement virtually identical to RA[5].

EPIDEMIOLOGY

Estimates of the prevalence of PsA among patients with psoriasis vary widely, with a widely accepted range of 6–42%[6,7]. Lack of a unified, validated definition of the disease coupled with the examination of heterogeneous populations may explain this broad estimate[2,8]. Nonetheless, research assessing disease prevalence reveals interesting trends. Northern European countries, for example, maintain higher prevalence of PsA than southern, a trend also found with skin disease. In a study from Sweden, for example, the prevalence of PsA in patients with psoriasis was 30%[9], roughly four times greater than that of an Italian study population with psoriasis[10] and twice that from a small sample of Croatian psoriatics[11]. Data aimed at assessing prevalence in the general population, rather than solely among patients with psoriasis, demonstrate similar latitudinal trends, with estimates of 1.1 cases per 1,000 in France[12] and 1.95 in Norway[13]. A rare study of incidence, or number of cases per unit time, revealed a rate of 23 cases per 100,000 per year in Finland[14].

In the United States, a recent population-based survey of psoriasis patients estimated prevalence of PsA at 11%[15]. As expected, incidence rates in America, estimated at around 6.6 cases per 100,000 per year, are less than a third of those in Finland[16].

The temporal relationship between the onset of skin and joint disease captures the attention of not only epidemiologists, but also clinical dermatologists. Data suggest that the vast majority of patients with PsA (80–90%) develop skin disease up to 10 years prior to arthritis, charging dermatologists with the task of continually assessing psoriatic patients for early evidence of joint pathology[17,18]. In 11–15% of patients, skin disease and arthritis commence simultaneously[5]. Rarely does joint disease present prior to skin involvement, except in the pediatric population, in which PsA prevalence may be grossly underestimated.

Other miscellaneous trends are noteworthy. Unlike RA, which maintains a strong female preponderance, PsA affects males and females equally[2,5,13]. The average age of onset ranges between 30 and 50 years[20]. Of the many phenotypes of psoriasis, plaque-type psoriatics are most likely to develop PsA[5].

GENETICS, IMMUNOLOGY, AND PATHOGENESIS

Studies of identical, or monozygotic, twins affirm the genetic basis of PsA (see also Chapter 1). Concordance rates vary between 35 and 70% among monozygotic twins and fall to 12–20% in dizygotic twins[4]. Other work suggests that first-degree relatives of those affected with PsA have a 50% greater risk of developing the disease than does the general population[20].

As with psoriasis, certain alleles encoding human leukocyte antigens (HLA), cellular glycoproteins involved with antigen presentation to T cells, associate with PsA. Class I loci, designated as HLA-A, -B, or -C, encode molecules that interact with CD8[+] T cells. Class II loci, HLA-D, encode peptides that interact with CD4[+] T cells. Certain polymorphisms of both class I and II alleles confer risk for PsA[21]. B-27, well known for its association with ankylosing spondylitis, in addition to B-17 and DR-4 maintain affiliation with PsA[22,23]. The well-described HLA-Cw 0602 allele, found in many patients with psoriatic skin disease, maintains only a moderate association with PsA[24,25].

Linkages studies, seeking association between the PsA phenotype and specific genetic loci, had been surprisingly fruitless initially. Indeed, early studies of the PSORS1 locus, tightly associated with psoriasis[26], failed to demonstrate linkage with PsA[27]. However, more recent genome-wide studies counter this by demonstrating association of various single nucleotide polymorphisms (SNPs) adjacent to PSORS1 with the PsA phenotype[25]. The PSORS2 locus on the long arm of chromosome 17, as well as loci encoding interleukin-12 and -23, have also demonstrated association with PsA[25,26,27].

Genetic differences in HLA molecules suggest that immune system dysregulation plays a significant role in the pathophysiology of PsA. Indeed, both the humoral and cellular systems are implicated. Serum and synovial fluid of PsA patients demonstrate increased immunoglobulins (Ig), particularly IgA and G[7,29]. To support the role of cellular immunity in PsA, activated CD8[+] T cells are prolific in synovial fluid[30]. Furthermore, medications preventing the activation of T cells have been a hallmark of treatment for PsA (see below).

CLINICAL MANIFESTATIONS

The distribution of affected joints, presence of psoriasis, and, in most cases, absence of rheumatoid factor characterize PsA. Radiological features, nail disease, and elements of the history also support the diagnosis. Patients with PsA often report a family history of psoriasis and/or psoriatic arthritis[31]. Classic symptoms of inflammatory arthritis can also lead the physician to the presence of PsA. Examples include morning joint stiffness lasting longer than 30 minutes that improves with activity, as well as arthralgias at rest[32].

Physical examination can point to PsA. Dactylitis (**250–252**), inflammation around an interphalangeal joint extending along an entire digit, strongly suggests PsA[31]. Another important sign, enthesitis (**253**), presents with tenderness at sites of insertion of ligaments and tendons. The examiner elicits pain on palpation of the Achilles region of the heel as well as ischial tuberosities and spinous processes. Nail disease (**254, 255**) particularly when adjacent to affected joints, may act as a marker for PsA. One study proposes that more than 20 nail pits may distinguish PsA from RA[33].

Clinical manifestations
250–252 Dactylitis. Swelling involves the entire digit and is most pronounced at the interphalangeal joint.
253 Enthesitis. Tenderness at the insertion of the Achilles tendon is common.
254, 255 Nail disease adjacent to affected joints.

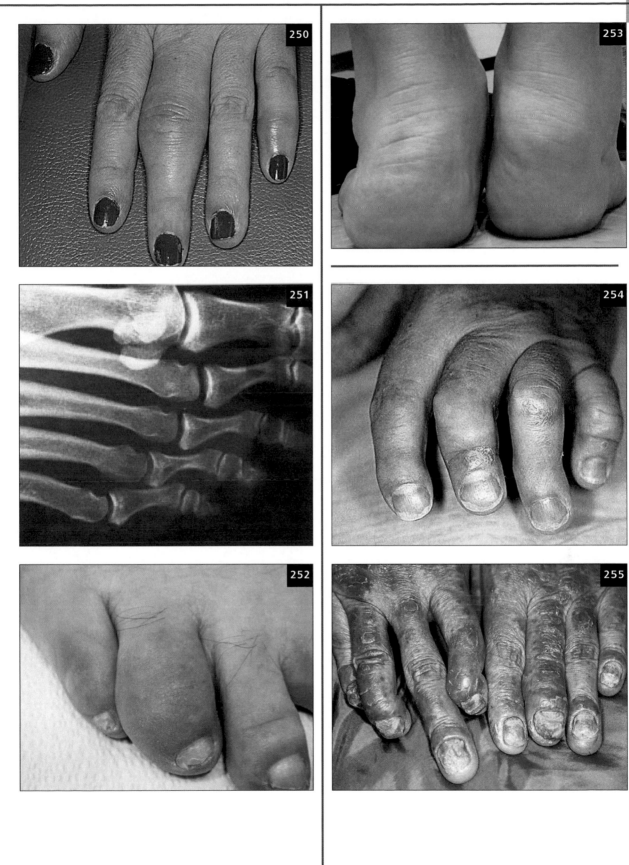

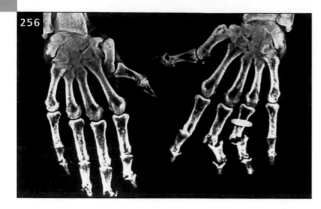

Clinical manifestations

256 Radiograph of PsA. Erosion of the DIP joints (acro-osteolysis) causing characteristic 'pencil-in-cup' deformity.
257 , 258 Asymmetric oligoarthritis.
259, 260 Symmetric polyarthritis.
261, 262 Distal interphalangeal (DIP) joint predominant. Note the adjacent nail disease.

Certain features of joint radiographs implicate PsA as well. The 'telescoping digits' of arthritis mutilans correspond radiographically with acro-osteolysis, termed 'pencil-in-cup' (**256**) deformity. Spine plain films in PsA demonstrate syndesmophytes, ossification of the outer layer of the intervertebral disk. In contrast to the 'bamboo spine' of ankylosing spondylitis, caused by circumferential ossification of consecutive disks, syndesmophytes in PsA are not symmetric or consecutive[5,34]. Other radiographic hallmarks include asymmetric inflammation of the sacroiliac joint and absence of bone loss adjacent to joints (so called 'juxta-articular osteopenia') typical of RA. Recent work suggests that MRI may be more sensitive in detecting clinically unapparent joint disease, including mild enthesitis[35].

Serum analysis aids little in the diagnosis and management of PsA. Despite classification as a 'seronegative' arthritis, 10–13% of patients are positive for RF[1].

Erythrocyte sedimentation rate (ESR), a non-specific marker of inflammation, correlates positively with measures of joint disability[36] and risk of death[37]. Another inflammatory marker, C reactive protein (CRP), may also be elevated[5].

With a disease as protean as PsA, problems arise with classification and diagnostic criteria. In the early 1970s, Moll and Wright described five subtypes of PsA (*Table 8*)[38]. The first, and reportedly most common, subtype is asymmetric oligoarthritis (**257, 258**). As the name implies, characteristic arthritis in fewer than five joints and lack of symmetry define this type of PsA. The next is symmetric polyarthritis, which affects metacarpal–phalangeal (MCP) joints symmetrically and resembles RA (**259, 260**). Arthritis involving the distal interphalangeal (DIP) joints predominantly characterizes the third subtype of PsA (**261, 262**). The fourth subtype is spondyloarthropathy, which tends to be asymmetric.

PsA subtype	Characteristics
Asymmetrical oligoarthritis	Commonest; predominantly peripheral; fewer than 5 joints; 'sausage'-like swelling (dactylitis).
Symmetric polyarthritis	Common; symmetric metacarpal–phalangeal joints; resembles rheumatoid arthritis
Predominant DIP joint involvement	Less common
Psoriatic spondylitis	Uncommon; predominantly axial; may involve sacroiliac joints
Arthritis mutilans	Uncommon; affects upto 10% of PsA patients; telescoping digits; destructive and debilitating

Table 8 Moll and Wright 1973 classification.
Characteristics of the five main subtypes of PsA.

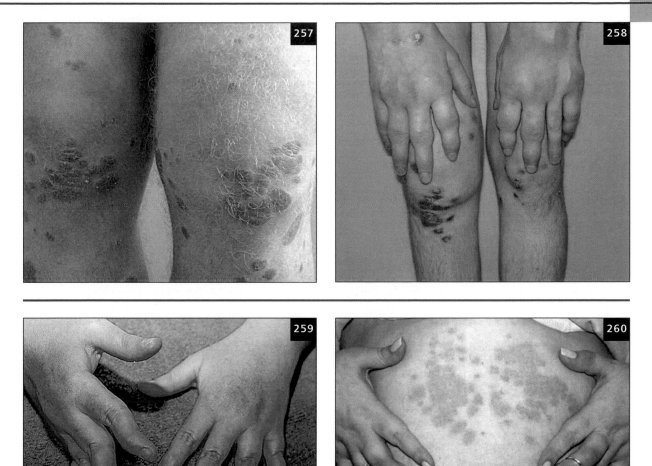

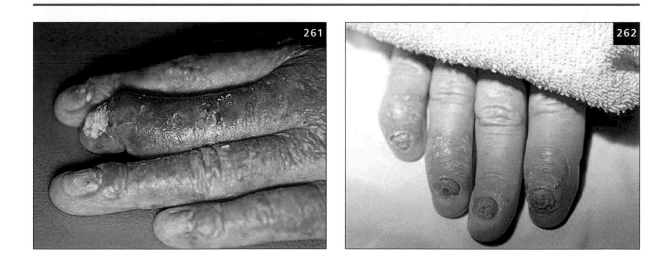

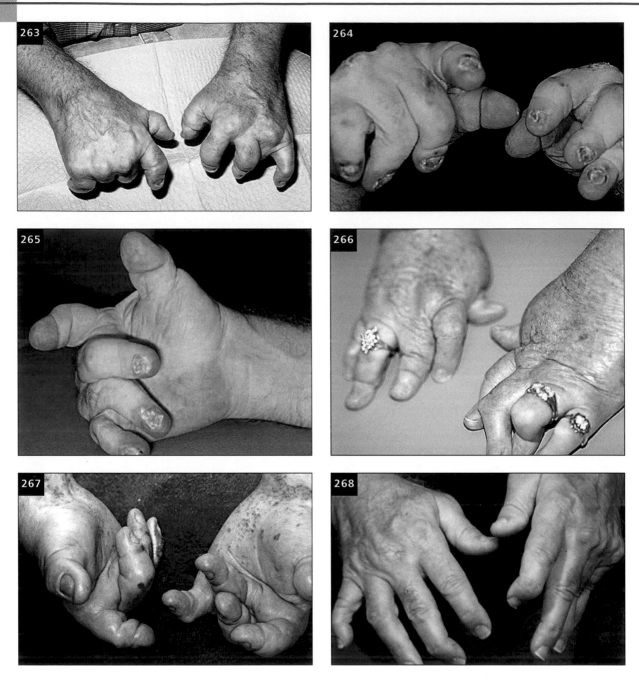

Clinical manifestations

263–268 Arthritis mutilans. Osteolysis of distal phalanges results in the characteristic 'telescoping' digits.

Arthritis mutilans (**263–268**), the destructive fifth subtype, may affect up to 10% of patients and can present with debilitating 'telescoping digits'[1]. Patients frequently suffer from more than one of the subtypes and, if inadequately treated, may progress from pauci to polyarticular arthritis and from erosive to osteolytic[39].

Many sets of diagnostic criteria for PsA exist, including those by Vasey and Espinoza[40], McGonagle *et al.*[41], Bennett[42], Moll and Wright[38], the European Spondyloarthropathy Study Group[43], and Gladman *et al.*[17]. In an effort to validate existing criteria, prominent rheumatologists undertook a large-scale international study, including 588 participants with PsA and 536 controls with other inflammatory arthritides[31]. The CASPAR (CIASsification criteria for PSoriatic Arthritis) study group recently determined that the criteria of Vasey and Espinoza were most sensitive (97%) and created a new criteria, highly sensitive (91.4%) and specific (98.7%) classification (*Table 9*).

The differential diagnosis of PsA is extensive. Clearly, evidence of current or prior psoriasis strongly suggests PsA in patients with arthralgias. However, pitfalls exist and, as stated above, joint disease may occasionally precede skin disease.

Key features differentiate PsA from similar forms of arthritis. RA may mimic some varieties of PsA, particularly the symmetric polyarthritis subtype described by Moll and Wright. However, features of RA such as female predominance, RF positivity, absence of spinal involvement, radiographic 'juxta-articular' erosions,

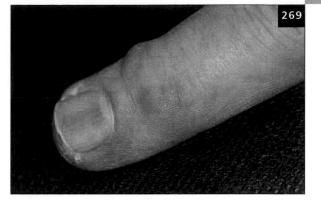

269

Clinical manifestations
269 Heberden's nodes, which can mimic the DIP joint deformity of PsA.

paucity of nail changes and absence of psoriatic skin changes distinguish it from PsA. RA may coexist with PsA in three per 100,000 cases[2].

Osteoarthritis (OA) may confuse the clinician suspecting DIP-joint predominant PsA. Heberden's nodes (**269**) – osteophytes at the DIP joint margins in OA – can mimic the joint deformity of PsA. Indeed, OA may be more common in psoriatics than in the general population, an effect likely mediated by a higher incidence of obesity[44]. However, important differences between OA and PsA exist. OA lacks features of inflammatory arthritis, for instance, as symptoms worsen with activity and are typically absent or mild in the morning[32].

CASPAR criteria
1 Evidence of current psoriasis, personal or family history of psoriasis
2 Typical psoriatic nail dystrophy: onycholysis, pitting, and hyperkeratosis
3 Negative rheumatoid factor
4 Current or history of dactylitis
5 Radiographic evidence of juxta-articular new bone formation (excluding osteophytes)

Table 9 CASPAR (classification criteria for psoriatic arthritis) criteria. For a diagnosis of PsA, patients should meet three out of these five criteria.

The variant of PsA involving the spine and sacrum overlaps with the other spondyloarthropathies. However, spinal inflammation in PsA is usually asymmetric and less debilitating than AS, for example[2]. Furthermore, spine radiographs of patients with AS demonstrate ossification of consecutive intervertebral disks, producing the characteristic 'bamboo spine,' whereas those of PsA tend to skip disks. As a result, PsA restricts the range of motion less than AS (**Table 10**).

PROGNOSIS

Research tracking outcomes demonstrates the toll PsA exacts on those affected. After following a cohort of patients with PsA for 20 years, one study revealed a 59% increase in mortality for women and a 65% increase for men compared to age-matched controls, although causes of death mirrored those of the general population[37]. Predictors of mortality included severity of joint disease, particularly erosion, as well as elevated ESR. More than five joints affected and 'high' dosages of medication, according to a different work, portend disease progression[45]. Females tend to progress more rapidly than males.

CONCLUSION

The identity of PsA lies not in a single blood test, clinical phenotype, or histological sample. Rather, a unique gestalt defines this disease, integrating a variety of clinical (rheumatological, as well as dermatological) and radiological manifestations, genetic and immunological markers, and epidemiologic trends. As such, PsA may represent an extension of all psoriatic disease: a unified whole that cannot be adequately described merely by the sum of its parts.

Table 10 **Differential diagnosis**. Differentiating qualities among psoriatic arthritis, rheumatoid arthritis, osteoarthritis, and ankylosing spondylitis[4].

Disease features	Psoriatic arthritis	Osteoarthritis	Ankylosing spondylitis	Rheumatoid arthritis
Morning stiffness in joints >30 minutes; improves with activity	Present	Absent	Present; especially vertebral	Present
Dactylitis	Present	Absent	Absent	Absent
Enthesitis	Present	Absent	Present	Absent
Pitting in adjacent nails	Present (>20 pits)	Absent	Absent	Occasionally present (<20 pits)
Gender predilection	None	Female > male	Male > female (3:1)	Female > male (3:1)
Radiological findings	Acral osteolysis ('pencil-in-cup' deformity), syndesmophytes not symmetric or consecutive, unilateral/asymmetric sacroiliitis	Osteophytes	Syndesmophytes; symmetric and consecutive, bridging of syndesmophytes ('bamboo spine') bilateral/symmetric sacroiliitis	Juxta-articular osteopenia
Rheumatoid factor	Usually negative (positive in 10–13%)	Negative	Negative	Positive
Associated HLA	Cw6	None	B27	DR4 (less commonly found in PsA)

5 | THERAPY

THE MANAGEMENT OF PSORIASIS must take into account not only the physical characteristics of the disease, i.e. number of plaques, body surface area (BSA) involvement (*270*), and phenotypical nature, but also the impact on the quality of life (QOL) of the patient. Thus, psoriasis involving localized areas, such as the palms and soles, while less than 5% of the total BSA, may produce a greater psychosocial impact than multiple patches on the trunk involving, say, 10% BSA.

MEASURING DISEASE

There are numerous measures of the physical extent of the disease: Psoriasis Area and Severity Index (PASI), Lattice Scale, Physician Global Assessment (PGA), and the Salford Psoriasis Index (SPI) (*Table 11*), while from a QOL perspective, the Dermatology Life Quality Index (DLQI) is the current standard. In addition, Short Form (SF)-36 and the Koo–Menter Psoriasis Instrument are less commonly used. See also Chapter 6 and Appendix. Finally, a new 'all-embracing' scoring index for psoriasis disability is being developed by the International Psoriasis Council, taking into account physical characteristics, quality of life issues, co-existent psoriatic joint disease, and a patient satisfaction index.

THERAPEUTIC OPTIONS

Treatment for psoriasis is commonly divided into (1) topical therapy, (2) phototherapy, and (3) systemic therapy, with topical therapy being utilized for the majority of patients, either as monotherapy or in combination with the other two classes of therapy[1]. This chapter reviews each of these three traditional approaches as well as the newest group of drugs – (4) biologic therapies – which target specific parts of the immune system.

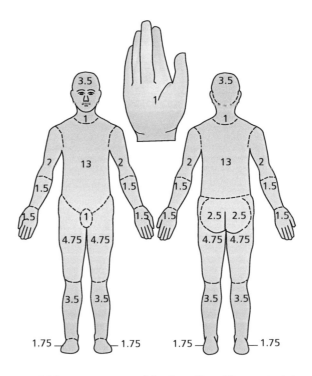

270 BSA. Measurement of the skin affected by psoriasis is described as a percentage of body surface area.

Measures of disease extent	
Physical	Psoriasis Area and Severity Index (PASI)
	Lattice scale
	Physician Global Assessment (PGA)
	Salford Psoriasis Index (SPI)
Quality of life	Dermatology Life Quality Index (DLQI)
	Short Form (SF)-36
	Koo–Menter Psoriasis Instrument (KMPI)

Table 11 Measures of disease extent. Quality of life parameters are as important as assessment of physical severity.

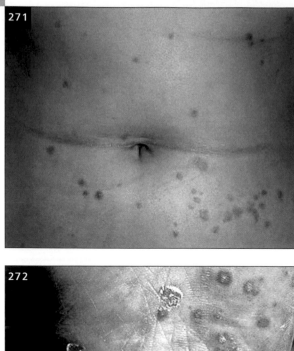

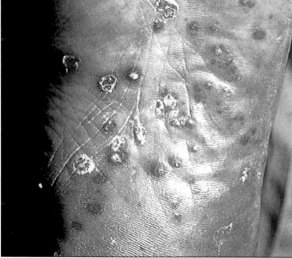

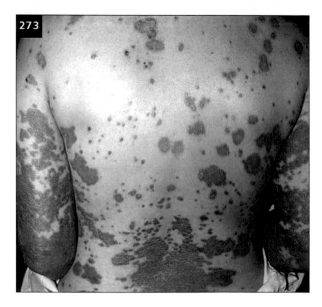

1 TOPICAL THERAPY

Topical therapy is the first line of defense in the treatment of mild-to-moderate psoriasis in the majority of patients, by reducing inflammation and excessive cell proliferation (271–273).

The nuances of topical therapy, e.g. amounts used, daily versus twice daily application, and side-effect profile, need to be discussed with all patients prior to initiating therapy. As compliance is frequently poor with topical therapy for a chronic disease like psoriasis, it is imperative that time be spent with patients on education and instruction. In addition, the absolute need to refrain from irritating the skin by rubbing, scratching, and picking, is critical, as well as the need to maintain adequate hydration of the skin with appropriate emollient creams, used especially after bathing and particularly in cold, dry seasons.

The spectrum of topical therapy for psoriasis is extremely broad, either as monotherapy or in combination with other topicals, phototherapy, and/or systemic therapy. In addition, each agent frequently has a wide spectrum of bases including creams, ointments, sprays, lotions, foams, and gels, particularly in the most commonly used group of agents, i.e. topical corticosteroids, necessitating the need for individualized therapy for each patient and body location (e.g. hairy versus non-hairy).

Topical corticosteroids

Fluorinated topical steroids have been available for psoriasis therapy for over 30 years. Corticosteroids are divided into different groups (*Table 12*) depending on their clinical efficacy and the vasoconstriction assay of Stoughton and Cornell[2,3]. The base of the topical steroid is targeted to the anatomical situation, e.g. foams, gels, and shampoos for the scalp; creams for thinner skin; and ointments for thicker skin, such as the elbows and knees.

Topical therapy
271 Amenable to topical therapy; limited disease.
272 May be amenable to topical therapy.
273 Not amenable to topical therapy.

Corticosteroid groups

Class 1	Very potent, up to 600 times as potent as hydrocortisone
Class 2	Potent, 150–100 times as potent as hydrocortisone
Class 3	Moderate, 2–25 times as potent as hydrocortisone
Class 4	Mild, hydrocortisone 0.5–2.5%

Table 12 Corticosteroid groups. This table shows the UK classification of four different potency classes. In the USA, a 7-potency rating is utlized[3,4].

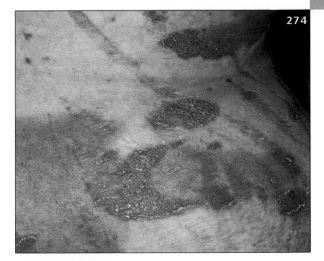

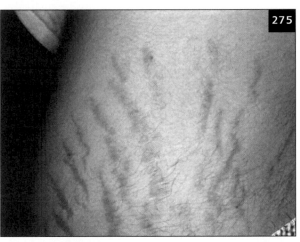

The very potent and potent topical steroid groups have been shown to have notable efficacy for psoriasis as compared to the mild and moderate potency agents. Thus, in the majority of cases, utilizing steroids within these two top groups will lead to significant clearing of psoriasis over a 4-week period. A major concern in the use of topical steroids and, hence, the restriction for the more potent agents to only short-term therapy, are local side-effects, such as atrophy, striae, purpura (**275, 276**) and telangiectases. Because of this, the potent and very potent topical steroids should never be used in flexures (breast folds, groin folds, axillae) or on the face (**277**).

Another side-effect of topical steroids is the induction of tolerance with ongoing therapy (tachyphylaxis), which occurs in a certain percentage of patients. Therefore, utilizing the more potent agents on an intermittent basis or on an interval basis, e.g. weekends only, may maintain the initial response while reducing cutaneous side-effects.

For extremely hypertrophic lesions, innovative approaches such as occluding potent topical steroids on a weekly basis may be highly effective.

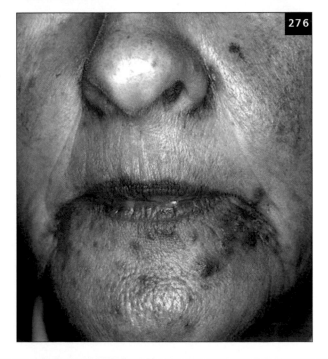

Local side-effects
274, 275 Striae.
276 Perioral dermatitis. An acneiform eruption may result from theuse of topical steroids on the face.

Vitamin D₃ derivatives

Currently three vitamin D_3 derivatives (calcitriol, tacalcitol, and calcipotriol), utilized for more than a decade, are available. As with topical steroids, they are available in a range of bases. Concerns regarding hypercalcemia as a result of excessive use of the agents, i.e. over 100 g per week, are reduced if the approved dosing schedules are utilized (*Table 13*). However, hypercalcemia secondary to overuse is extremely uncommon.

The major benefit of this group of agents is its lack of steroid-related side-effects, as discussed above. The only significant side-effect profile is the potential for irritation, stinging, and burning, which occurs in approximately up to a third of patients. Therefore, as with corticosteroids, this group should be used cautiously in flexures and on the face. As monotherapy, these agents are equivalent in potency to low to mid-potency topical steroids[4,5]. Many innovative schedules utilizing vitamin D_3 preparations in combination with potent or very potent topical steroids have been utilized, including induction regimens with topical steroids for 2 weeks and thereafter adding vitamin D_3 derivatives from Monday to Friday, with weekend use of the potent topical steroids (pulse therapy).

In order to improve patient compliance – a major issue with twice-daily usage of topical agents and/or innovative weekend-type programs as discussed above – a new topical agent utilized on a once-daily basis has been developed, containing the potent topical steroid betamethasone dipropionate plus vitamin D_3 in a single stable preparation. These two products cannot be compounded extemporaneously due to pH differences; however, the combination product now available as Dovobet® and Daivobet® in Europe and Taclonex® in the United States has been shown to maintain efficacy with minimal side-effects from each of the two active ingredients over a 1-year course of treatment[6]. However, it does not give the rapid initial response of the ultrapotent corticosteroids.

Calcineurin inhibitors

The two main agents in this group are pimecrolimus and tacrolimus, commonly used in the treatment of atopic dermatitis. Because of concerns regarding topical steroid and vitamin D_3 usage in sensitive areas, e.g. flexures and face, these two agents have been studied in psoriasis therapy for these areas. Recent studies have shown they are very effective for inverse and facial psoriasis[7,8], but of limited value in psoriasis elsewhere on the body.

Table 13 Vitamin D₃ analogs used for the treatment of psoriasis. Using more than the recommended dosage may increase the risk of hypercalcemia.

[Excerpted from Menter A, Griffiths CEM (2007). Current and future management of psoriasis. Lancet; 370: 272–284, with permission]

Monotherapy or in combination	Vehicles available	Maximum recommended dosage per week
Calcitriol 3 µg/g	Ointment	210 g
Tacalcitol 4 µg/g	Ointment	70 g
Calcipotriol 50 µg/g*	Cream, ointment, scalp solution	100 g of cream or ointment, 60 ml of scalp solution
Calcipotriol 50 µg/g + betamethasone dipropionate 0.5 mg/g	Ointment	100 g

*Generic name in the USA is calcipotriene.

Topical tazarotene

This derivative of vitamin A, available in gel or cream formulations in concentrations of 0.05% or 0.1%, has been utilized for psoriasis for over a decade; however, it is only modestly effective. A significant concern is the irritancy potential, usually perilesional (**277, 278**), so caution is advised when utilizing this therapy, usually only once daily to minimize the risk. To further reduce the irritancy potential of tazarotene, this agent is frequently used in combination with topical steroids, i.e. topical tazarotene at night, carefully applied and rubbed in completely, together with use of a topical steroid by day[9]. Due to the potential for systemic absorption when used over widespread areas of the body, and the known teratogenicity of systemic tazarotene, this agent should not be used during pregnancy.

Dithranol (anthralin) and coal tar preparations

These two agents have been used for over a century in the treatment of psoriasis, usually in combination with phototherapy. Goeckerman, in 1921, first introduced the use of tar and phototherapy at the Mayo Clinic[10] (see p.45). Ingram, in 1948, then introduced the combination of dithranol and phototherapy in Leeds[11]. Both of these agents are again available in multiple bases, such as ointments, pastes, shampoos, and solutions. The cosmetic unacceptability of these two products has limited their use to predominantly outpatient specialized treatment centers. To limit the significant irritancy and staining potential of dithranol, it is frequently employed in a 'short contact' fashion for periods of up to 1 hour before removal. Tar preparations are frequently used in shampoos for scalp involvement, but very few clinical studies have shown durable responses (**279**).

The use of both these products has been waning, particularly with the introduction of the newer vitamin D3 preparations, with equal or greater efficacy and less irritancy.

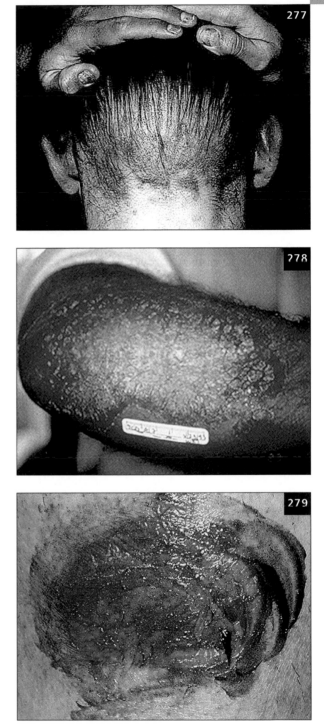

Topical therapy
277, 278 Tazarotene perilesional irritation.
279 Irritancy and staining potential with tars and, particularly, anthralin.

2 PHOTOTHERAPY AND PUVA

Ultraviolet light therapy, natural and artificial, has been utilized in the treatment of psoriasis for centuries. In the eighteenth and nineteenth centuries, artificial UV light sources first became available for therapeutic usage including the treatment of tuberculosis and psoriasis.

The ultraviolet light spectrum, which extends from 200 to 400 nm, is divided arbitrarily into three main regions based on wavelength: (1) 200–290 nm, ultraviolet light C, predominantly has germicidal effects; (2) 290–320 nm, ultraviolet light B, broadband, predominantly used for the treatment of psoriasis, with a narrow 311–313 nm wavelength the most effective (narrowband UVB); and (3) 320–400 nm, UVA, predominantly used for psoriasis therapy in combination with topical and systemic photosensitizers, such as methoxsalen (8-methoxypsoralen) (see below).

Mechanism of action

It is likely that phototherapy, both broadband and more specifically the narrowband wavelengths, has a direct effect on cytokine production by both TH1 and TH2 T-cell populations, as well as potentially changing antigen-presenting cell activity and having direct effects on natural killer cell activity. The result is a broad-based downregulation of cell-mediated immune function with subsequent benefits for psoriasis[12].

Broadband UVB (BB-UVB)

In broadband UVB, the predominant light source utilized is fluorescent UVB bulbs, which consist of a low-pressure mercury discharge source enclosed in a long glass tube coated with a phosphor. Upon electrical stimulation, the mercury vapor emits 254-nm radiation, which excites the phosphor coating to emit energies of longer wavelength, with wavelength emission dependent on the type of phosphor 'coating.' These tubes may be of different lengths, i.e. 4 foot (120 cm) and 6 foot (180 cm) utilized in individual panels or in specific cabinets in dermatology clinics.

Absolute exclusion criteria
Erythroderma
History of multiple skin cancers
History of photosensitive disorders, e.g. lupus erythematosus
History of photoaggravated psoriasis
Relative exclusion criteria
Prior exposure to ionizing radiation or arsenic
Family history of melanoma or other skin cancers
Severe actinic damage
Flexural psoriasis

Table 14 **Exclusion criteria for UVB phototherapy**[13].

History
Topical and systemic medication use
Melanoma and skin cancer history
Cardiovascular instability
Light-sensitive disorders
Information provided to patients
Activities required before each session
Expected experiences during treatment
General compliance requirements to optimize therapy
Cost and insurance considerations
Warnings
UVB keratitis if goggles are not used (throughout treatment)
Potential to develop skin cancer
'Burning' of skin
Itching and dryness of skin
Potential for reactivation of herpes simplex infection
Possibility of treatment failure
Information and instructions for patients
Use of topical preparations before and after each session
Avoidance of additional exposure to sunlight or other UV source
Consultation with treatment center physician before initiating new prescriptions or over-the-counter products
Prohibition of other therapies unless approved by the treatment center physician
Projected number of treatments required for remission and maintenance

Table 15 **Patient information.** Checklist required before initiating UVB phototherapy.

Candidates for all forms of phototherapy are predominantly patients with moderate degrees of psoriasis, particularly guttate and small plaque psoriasis. Patients with larger, more hypertrophic or lichenified plaques of psoriasis are not candidates, unless the therapy is combined with other agents such as systemic retinoids (see below). In addition, patients unresponsive to topical therapy, with more widespread disease, may be considered for phototherapy.

Exclusion criteria are outlined in **Table 14** and the checklist to be followed before initiating UVB phototherapy is given in **Table 15**.

Dosing schedule for UVB phototherapy

It is imperative that the output of the UVB light inside the phototherapy unit be checked on a regular, e.g. monthly, basis[13]. This reading is normally given in milliwatts per centimeter squared (mW/cm^2). The initial dose is determined by virtue of the patient's skin type (**Table 16**).

Treatment is normally given three to four times weekly, with dosage increments based either on skin type, i.e. 5 mJ/cm^2 increase for type I and 25–30 mJ/cm^2 for type VI, pending no significant erythema with the prior treatment, or based on minimum erythema dosage (MED), which is determined at the first visit, with subsequent increases by 10–25% of this MED at each visit. Generally speaking, approximately 20–25 treatments are required for significant clearing of widespread, small plaque psoriasis. However, inevitably, psoriasis will tend to slowly return and, hence, maintenance schedules are frequently employed, e.g. once- weekly or even twice-monthly. Adjunctive topical therapy for face, scalp, and flexures is usually required due to the inability of phototherapy to clear these areas.

Narrowband UVB (NB-UVB)

This specialized TL-01 lamp emits a narrow band of high-intensity UVB light of between 311 and 313 nm. This was shown to be the wavelength of choice for psoriasis patients by John Parrish and colleagues in Boston in 1981[14]. Whereas the majority of dermatologists in Europe have converted from broadband (BB) to narrowband (NB), the opposite is the case in the United States, where phototherapy is not as frequently utilized. Initial dosing of narrowband UVB is based on the patient's MED; thus, the initial dose given is 50% of the MED, with subsequent dose increments of approximately 10–20% of the MED. Alternatively, dosing can be based on skin type, i.e. skin type I with an initial narrowband UVB dose of 300 mJ/cm^2, increasing to approximately 600–800 mJ/cm^2 for skin types V and VI, with approximately 100 mJ/cm^2 increase with subsequent dosing. The cost of replacement bulbs for NB-UVB is distinctly higher than for BB-UVB.

Response with NB therapy is superior to BB-UVB[15], although it may not be quite as effective as PUVA[16]. From a safety perspective at this stage, it appears that NB-UVB has not shown any increase in carcinogenesis over broadband UVB in humans, although tests in mouse models suggested that TL-01 NB-UVB light sources are two to three times more carcinogenic per MED dose than BB-UVB[17].

Due to ease of administration, lack of need for prior oral or topical photoactive agent, and safety history to date, NB-UVB has significantly reduced the use of PUVA, although the latter remains more efficacious. In a 1999 study of 100 patients, PUVA therapy given twice weekly was more effective than NB-UVB, with a significant reduction in the number of treatments required for clearing and with longer remissions[18].

Table 16 **Dosing guidelines for broadband UVB.**

Skin type	Typical features	Tanning ability	Initial UVB dose	UVB increase after each treatment
Type I	Very pale skin, blue/hazel eyes	Always burns, never tans	20 mJ/cm^2	5 mJ/cm^2
Type II	Fair skin, blue eyes	Burns easily, rarely tans	25 mJ/cm^2	10 mJ/cm^2
Type III	Darker white skin	Tans after initial burn	30 mJ/cm^2	15 mJ/cm^2
Type IV	Light brown skin	Burns occasionally, tans readily	40 mJ/cm^2	20 mJ/cm^2
Type V	Brown skin	Rarely burns, tans readily	50 mJ/cm^2	25 mJ/cm^2
Type VI	Dark brown or black skin	Never burns, always tans	60 mJ/cm^2	30 mJ/cm^2

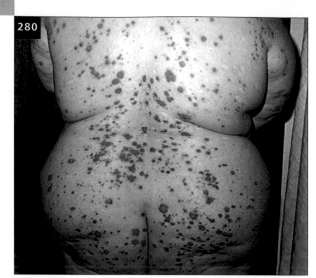

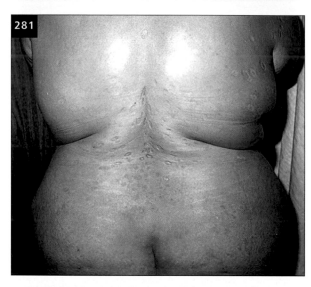

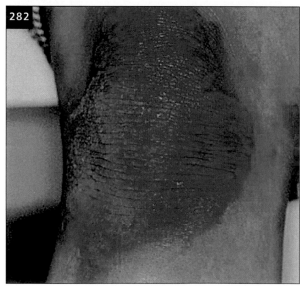

Combination therapy

280 Pre-Goeckerman treatment.
281 Post-Goeckerman treatment.
282 Staining as a result of Ingram dithranol (anthralin) therapy.

UVB combination therapy

On occasion, patients may be treated with both UVA and UVB radiation, particularly patients on PUVA therapy who are showing a less than optimal response to treatment and are at the upper limit of dosing for UVA[19].

The most commonly used phototherapy combination is with low-dose (approximately 10 mg/day) systemic retinoids, i.e. acitretin, in combination with PUVA therapy. Ideally, the retinoids are initiated approximately 2 weeks prior to initiation of PUVA therapy. Systemic retinoids may also be used very effectively with narrow-band UVB, again with significant improvement likely[19]. Topical retinoids, e.g. tazarotene, may also be utilized for thinning of more hypertrophic plaques to reduce the number and dose of PUVA therapies given.

Goeckerman therapy

In 1925, William Goeckerman at the Mayo Clinic developed a combination therapy using hot quartz mercury vapor lamps, together with all-day and night immersion of patients' psoriasis plaques in crude coal-tar preparations[11]. This hospital regimen has subsequently been shortened to a 6–8-hour day-care regimen in a few specialized centers internationally, with excellent results and long (up to 6 months) remissions (**280, 281**)[20].

Ingram regimen

In 1953, Professor John Ingram in Leeds introduced the combination of dithranol (anthralin) subsequent to UVB therapy, with significantly better response than with UVB therapy alone[10]. However, as discussed previously, dithranol's irritation and staining have led to a reduction in the use of this combination therapy (**282**).

Targeted phototherapy

More recently, a new excimer laser has been introduced for the treatment of psoriasis. This uses a 308-nm xenon chloride light source to treat individual plaques of psoriasis, initially three times weekly, with an average of approximately 10–12 treatments normally required for improvement. Thus, a significant reduction of radiation and even of number of treatments required may be seen

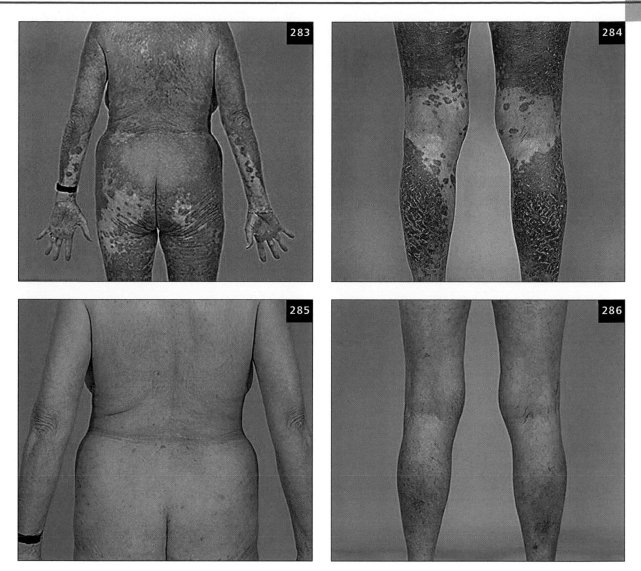

PUVA therapy
283, 284 Pre-therapy.
285, 286 Post-therapy.

for localized skin involvement[21]. As with all forms of therapy, caution needs to be exercised relating to blistering, burning, and even pain when using the excimer laser, with another potential side-effect being post-inflammatory hyperpigmentation subsequent to clearance of individual plaques. In a recent study evaluating the excimer laser in comparison with a pulse-dye laser, a higher response was noted with the excimer laser, although a subset of patients did respond better with the pulse-dye laser[22]. Long-term remissions lasting 3 months to 1 year were seen with both lasers.

PUVA therapy

In 1974, Drs John Parrish, Tom Fitzpatrick, and colleagues in Boston published the first paper on the use of oral methoxsalen and long-wave ultraviolet light in the *New England Journal of Medicine*. They showed that 21 adult Caucasian patients with generalized psoriasis, with at least 50% of the body involved, had complete clearance of psoriatic lesions in comparison with conventional ultraviolet light therapy (**283–286**)[23]. This was followed by a cooperative study in 1977 in which 1,308 patients were treated two to three times weekly with oral 8-methoxypsoralen followed by UVA photo-therapy. Major clearance occurred in 88% of these patients, over a course of 18–20 treatments[24]. More recently, 5-methoxypsoralen (5-MOP) has been introduced as the photosensitizing agent of choice versus 8-methoxypsoralen (8-MOP), due to the lower incidence of gastrointestinal side-effects – predominantly nausea and vomiting – commonly seen with 8-MOP.

Great caution must be exercised to prevent photo-toxicity, i.e. redness, itching, and sunburn with PUVA and a careful drug history must always be taken to limit photosensitivity secondary to oral medications. Thus, close monitoring of patients at each visit is essential, together with total body evaluations at intervals for evidence of new actinic keratosis, squamous cell carcinomas, atypical nevi, etc. It appears that the lesion clearance rates are equivalent with 5-MOP and 8-MOP given approximately 1 hour prior to UVA irradiation. One of the significant benefits of PUVA therapy, in addition to excellent clearance rates, is the duration of remissions, with 6-month remissions not uncommon following a single course of treatment. However, side-effects relating to PUVA therapy must be carefully considered, particularly photocarcinogenesis, with increasing rates of squamous cell carcinoma seen, predominantly after a total of 250 PUVA treatments over an individual's lifetime have been given, thus restricting its long-term continuous usage[25,26]. In addition to squamous cell carcinoma, there is a potential increase in melanoma which has been noted in the original cohort of 1,308 PUVA patients carefully followed up by Robert Stern *et al.*[26] over the past 30 years. There is also a significant risk of cutaneous photo-aging and an increased number of benign yet unsightly lentigines seen in patients with long-term PUVA therapy. There are a number of contraindications to PUVA therapy including patients with photosensitivity disorders, such as lupus erythematosus, as well as in immunosuppressed patients due to increased risk of skin cancer. Caution also needs to be exercised in patients with extensive solar damage and a history of multiple skin cancers. PUVA is extremely valuable in thick-plaque psoriasis and in those failing to respond to traditional UVB therapy, as well as in patients of skin types III and above who are less at risk of photo-aging and skin cancer than lighter-skinned patients. In addition to recalcitrant psoriasis, PUVA therapy may frequently benefit the palms

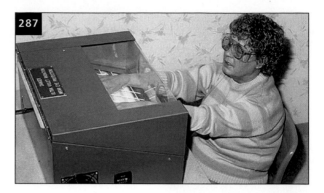

Topical PUVA therapy.
287 A small unit for hand/foot treatment. Eye protection is essential during PUVA therapy.

288 Full-body combination UVB/PUVA unit.

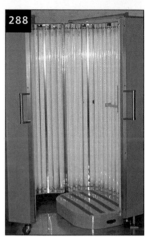

and soles, especially when given topically, i.e. immersion of the localized areas with a topical psoralen mixture applied pre-UVA exposure. Caution needs to be taken when utilizing this to prevent burns (**287, 288**)[27].

It is absolutely essential that eye protection be utilized during PUVA therapy, in addition to the standard protection of face and genitalia. Patients also need to wear protective UVA-blocking glasses when outdoors, in a vehicle, or even when close to a window, for approximately 18 hours subsequent to PUVA therapy. Provided these precautions are rigidly adhered to, risk of cataract formation is no higher than in the general population. However, yearly ophthalmologic evaluation is recommended.

Without the use of oxsoralen prior to UVA exposure, light sources, as used in a tanning salon as monotherapy, show only moderate response[28].

3 TRADITIONAL SYSTEMIC THERAPY

The rationale for systemic therapy is summarized in *Table 17*. Patients are candidates for phototherapy or systemic therapy when their psoriasis is more widespread, disabling, or creates significant impairment in quality of life (QOL) (**289**) (see also p.115). The exact choice of therapy in these situations requires considerable physician judgment. In addition, work schedules or other obligations may preclude compliance with a phototherapy regimen. Other factors, such as ethanol use, past cumulative doses of methotrexate or ciclosporin, a history of hypertension, or family planning issues, may influence decisions about the ideal treatment for any particular patient.

289 Diagnostic algorithm. Criteria to determine if a psoriasis patient is a candidate for systemic treatment or phototherapy. *Note that phototherapy (including forms of UVB and PUVA treatment) can be used for the treatment of psoriasis skin lesions in patients with psoriatic arthritis, but these patients will also require systemic treatment for the coexistent joint involvement. Patients with significant psoriatic arthritis will require systemic therapy.

Table 17 The rationale for systemic therapy.

Reasons for systemic therapy I

Poor or no response to, or impractical to consider:
- Topical therapy
- UVB Phototherapy
- Photochemotherapy (PUVA)

Received maximum 'safe' cumulative PUVA dose

Reasons for systemic therapy II

Psoriasis covers more than 10% of the body surface area (BSA; 1% is palm-sized)

Severe inflammatory forms of psoriasis:
- Generalized pustular psoriasis
- Erythrodermic psoriasis

Reasons for systemic therapy III

Physical restrictions:
- Incapacitating hand or foot psoriasis
- Associated psoriatic joint disease
- Psoriasis precluding gainful employment

Negative impact on quality of life (QOL):
- Social and personal interactions
- Severe emotional distress

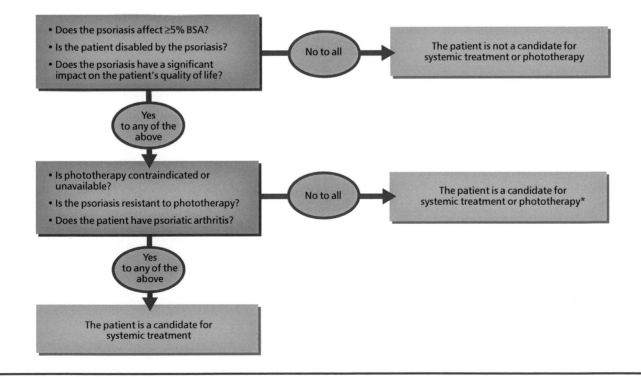

Dermatologists are fortunate in having a wide array of systemic therapies available, i.e. traditional agents and biological agents. Traditionally, systemic therapy has been reserved for patients with moderate-to-severe psoriasis. Definitions relating to moderate-to-severe are frequently based on body surface area (BSA) involvement, i.e. 0–5% mild psoriasis, 5–10% moderate psoriasis, >10% more severe involvement. However, as can be seen from *Table 11* (p.81), a number of other issues relating to QOL considerations must also be assessed:

- Does the patient have more than 5% BSA involvement?
- Is the patient disabled by psoriasis?
- Does the psoriasis have a significant impact on the patient's quality of life?
- Is phototherapy contraindicated or not reasonably feasible for the patient?
- Is the psoriasis resistant to phototherapy?
- Does the patient have psoriatic arthritis?

Recently an index, the Koo–Menter Psoriasis Instrument (KMPI) has been devised to help physicians identify candidates for systemic therapy. This is an assessment tool that dermatologists can readily use in their daily practice. It provides an assessment of psoriasis-specific health-related quality of life (HRQOL), using a 12-part questionnaire filled out by patients. Thereafter, the physician reviews the locations and extent of the disease, as well as the presence or absence of psoriatic joint disease. Thus, physicians can evaluate quality of life, disease severity, and disability, and make recommendations for potential systemic therapy. Despite the multiple systemic agents available for therapy, patients with moderate-to-severe psoriasis are frequently undertreated. For example, 87% of patients with severe psoriasis receive topical therapy and only approximately 27% of these patients have ever tried methotrexate[29], a drug which in some parts of the world is underutilized, e.g. only half the dermatologists in the United States have prescribed methotrexate for psoriasis[30].

Traditional agents
METHOTREXATE (MTX)

Formally approved for the treatment of psoriasis in 1971, methotrexate is still considered the gold standard for the treatment of psoriasis worldwide. Thus, as the first systemic antipsoriatic therapy introduced, it continues to play a major role in the management of psoriasis. Methotrexate is a competitive inhibitor of the enzyme dihydrofolate reductase, inhibiting pyrimidine and purine nucleotides, essential for rapidly dividing cells, e.g. epidermal keratinocytes. In the initial year of use of methotrexate, different schemata were devised based on epidermal cell cycle turnover, e.g. three doses per week every 12 hours over a 24-hour period. However, more recent work has verified the specific effect that methotrexate has on T-lymphocytes, which is likely to be the primary focus of methotrexate's benefit in psoriasis, with epidermal cell proliferation a secondary effect. Methotrexate is normally initiated in doses of 7.5–15 mg per week, given either as a single dose or divided into three 12-hourly dosages. Pending clinical response, the dose may be slowly titrated up to 25 mg, or even 30 mg per week. Few randomly controlled trials are available for methotrexate, the first being a study comparing methotrexate and ciclosporin over the course of 16 weeks of treatment[31]. Essentially an open-label study (with no placebo arm), this trial showed that 60% of treated patients with moderate-to-severe psoriasis attained a PASI 75 score at the end of the 16-week period. A more recent study, the CHAMPION study, was the first to compare methotrexate with a known biological agent, adalimumab, and, importantly, a placebo. In this multicenter European study, only 37% of methotrexate-treated patients attained the PASI 75 score at the end of 16 weeks. This study may have underestimated the efficacy of methotrexate, as the initial 'starting' dose was low (7.5 mg/week) with limitation of the subsequent dose escalation after 8 weeks and the attainment of PASI 50 during the course of the study.

Contraindications

Contraindications
Decreased renal function
Abnormal baseline liver function test or history of hepatitis
Male/female fertility
Severe anemia, leucopenia, or thrombocytopenia
Excess alcohol consumption
Active infections
Unreliable patient
Obesity
Diabetes

Table 18 Contraindications to methotrexate.
These include renal dysfunction and liver disease.

Drug interactions
NSAIDs
All nephrotoxins
Sulfonamides and derivatives*
Penicillins and cephalosporins
Colchicine and probenicid
Barbiturates and dilantin

*Bactrim® and Septra®

Table 19 Methotrexate drug interactions.
Concomitant administration of methotrexate with NSAIDs
can cause bone marrow suppression, while penicillin may
affect renal clearance.

Risk factors for liver disease
Excess alcohol consumption
History of liver disease/abnormal liver function tests
Intravenous drug abuse
Diabetes
Obesity
Previous exposure to hepatotoxic drugs
Hepatitis B and C

Table 20 Risk factors for liver disease. Methotrexate is
hepatotoxic with long-term use.

Contraindications to methotrexate

The most important side-effects of methotrexate relate
to bone marrow suppression, particularly in patients
with poor renal function or when the drug is inadver-
tently combined with certain medications such as sulfonamides and other anti-inflammatory agents (**Tables
18, 19**). Therefore, the complete blood count is monitored. In addition, folic acid supplementation is now
routinely used to avoid folic acid deficiency and reduce
the risk of hepatotoxicity and the incidence of other negative side-effects (see below). The other important risk
factor to be considered when initiating methotrexate
therapy is that of liver disease. Risk factors for liver
disease need to be carefully assessed before initiating
therapy and patients counseled accordingly, particularly
relating to excess alcohol consumption and concomitant medication usage (**Table 20**).

Other side-effects relating to methotrexate include
gastrointestinal upset, i.e. nausea, vomiting, as well as
fatigue and headaches, often lasting 24–48 hours post
dosing on a weekly basis.

Monitoring for bone marrow suppression and liver toxicity

Monthly monitoring of complete blood count is essential. Particularly in elderly patients with decreased renal
function tests, periodic assessment of kidney function
must take place. At each visit, patients should be ques-
tioned about dry, persistent, nonproductive cough,
which could potentially be a symptom of methotrexate-
induced pneumonitis, a rare but important side-effect.
Both males and females need to be counseled relating to
pregnancy, with 3-month wait time strongly advised for
both men and women post-completion of methotrexate
before considering conception and pregnancy.

Liver toxicity

As with bone marrow toxicity, liver function tests are
assessed at regular intervals. A major cause for debate is
the recommendation for liver biopsy; new American
Academy of Dermatology guidelines (2009) on the use
of methotrexate in psoriasis have raised the threshold for
biopsy to a cumulative dose of 3.5–4 g, i.e. after approximately 5–7 years of continuous therapy[32]. The need for
liver biopsy continues to be reduced with the advent of
the procollagen IIIA serological test, now in common
use in Europe, and pending new scanning tools for
screening of liver fibrosis (see also p.122)[33,34].

Liver biopsies

Liver biopsies are graded on a I–IV basis, with grade IIIA changes equating to mild fibrosis, grade IIIB changes equating to moderate-to-severe fibrosis, and grade IV equaling liver cirrhosis. Thus, patients with grades IIIB or IV changes need to be discontinued from further methotrexate therapy[35].

Treatment with methotrexate, as discussed earlier, remains a very important systemic therapy for moderate-to-severe psoriasis, with major benefits being its low cost and ready availability compared to other systemic agents. In combination with biologic agents, low-dose (7.5–12.5 mg weekly) methotrexate provides additional benefits in terms of preservation and augmentation of therapeutic response of both psoriasis and psoriatic arthritis with minimal/no additional side-effects or drug interactions. Provided patients are carefully selected and carefully monitored on a routine basis, methotrexate must still be considered as a first-choice treatment in patients in this category.

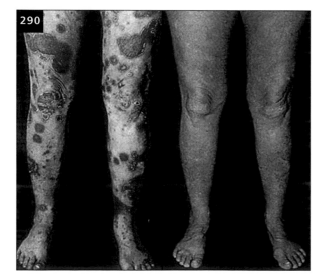

290 Traditional agents. Pre- and post-ciclosporin therapy.

CICLOSPORIN

Ciclosporin (CyA) was first noted to benefit psoriasis in 1979[36], subsequent to which multiple clinical studies have verified its efficacy, particularly in short-term therapy for patients with moderate-to-severe psoriasis. Ciclosporin's function is dependent on its binding to cyclophilin, resulting in further binding of the ciclosporin–cyclophilin complex to calcineurin phosphatase, which leads to blocking of T-cell activation. It is normally utilized in a dose of 2.5–5 mg/kg per day, with multiple clinical studies underscoring its significant clinical efficacy, particularly when used in short-term, i.e. 12–16 weeks, courses. Thus, the majority of patients get significant improvement, both in clinical, as well as quality of life measurements[37–39] (**290**).

This drug has been approved in the United States for 1-year continuous therapy, with prior approval in Europe for 2 years of continuous therapy. However, it is best used as a short-term, i.e. 12–16-week, course of treatment to produce rapid, if not complete, clearing of disease in the majority of patients. Remissions, as with methotrexate, are approximately 3–4 months in duration[40]. Thus, in the majority of cases, treatment can commence at 2.5–3.0 mg/kg taken in two divided doses, with dose adjustments of approximately 0.5 mg/kg up to a maximum of 5.0 mg/kg per day, with onset of action normally seen within 2 weeks of initiation. As with methotrexate, dosing monitoring, side-effects, and drug interactions with ciclosporin are critical.

Ciclosporin dosing and monitoring

Ciclosporin dosing and monitoring involve:

- Careful dermatological and physical examination.
- Blood pressure measurement (on two separate occasions at baseline).
- Laboratory tests:
  – Serum creatinine (on two occasions)
  – Blood urea nitrogen (BUN)
  – Complete blood count (CBC)
  – Uric acid
  – Liver function tests
  – Lipids and electrolytes (including magnesium)
  – Urinalysis.
- Meticulous verbal (and written) instructions regarding the nature and implementation of CyA therapy monitoring and drug interactions should be given to patients.

Ciclosporin side-effects

Common side-effects are renal insufficiency and hypertension, while less frequent ones are liver toxicity, hypertrichosis, gingival hyperplasia, acne, and neuropathy.

Ciclosporin drug interactions

Many drugs can interact with ciclosporin; they include sulfonamides, erythromycins, ketoconazole, trimethoprim, barbiturates, nonsteroidal anti-inflammatory drugs, and probenecid.

The main recommendations for the use of ciclosporin in the management of psoriasis are outlined in *Ciclosporin in Psoriasis Clinical Practice: An International Consensus Statement*[41] as follows:

- Intermittent short courses (average of 12 weeks duration) of ciclosporin are preferable.
- Ciclosporin should be given in the dose range 2.5–5.0 mg/kg per day.
- Treatment regimens tailored to the needs of patients.
- Psychosocial disability, as well as clinical extent of disease and failure of previous treatment, should be taken into account.
- Renal function should be assessed before and during treatment.
- Adherence to treatment guidelines substantially reduces the risk of adverse events.
- Long-term continuous ciclosporin therapy may be appropriate in a subgroup of patients; duration should be kept below 2 years whenever possible.
- When long-term continuous ciclosporin therapy is necessary, annual evaluation of glomerular filtration rate may be useful to accurately monitor renal function.

Thus, it is critical to monitor renal function, as well as blood pressure, as ciclosporin therapy causes vasoconstriction of the renal arterioles, leading to a decrease in glomerular filtration rate. Guidelines recommend that, should the serum creatinine increase by 25–30% above baseline, the dose of ciclosporin should be reduced or even discontinued, suggesting that the optimal use of this drug is short intermittent courses, allowing 'drug holidays' for normalization of renal function studies. However, in young, healthy patients, longer treatment periods of up to 1–2 years may be undertaken before considering alternative therapies. Those with pre-existing renal disease, those with hypertension, and elderly patients need to be carefully screened and, if necessary, alternative therapeutic methods utilized.

As ciclosporin is an immunosuppressive agent, it is important to monitor patients for cancer, particularly skin cancer. Patients with a prior history of PUVA therapy are at significant risk for nonmelanoma skin cancer, i.e. squamous cell carcinoma, particularly with maintenance of ciclosporin therapy over a 1 to 2-year period[42]. It is unclear whether ciclosporin leads to increased systemic neoplasms, with the results of a long-term study – > 2 years cumulative treatment – failing to reveal any higher risk[42].

Weekly to bimonthly screening for patients on ciclosporin therapy should include:
- Blood pressure weekly to twice monthly.
- Serum creatinine every 2 weeks for the first 2 months, thereafter monthly.
- Serum lipids and serum magnesium at infrequent intervals, i.e. two or three times yearly.
- Drug interactions:
  – Drugs increasing nephrotoxicity, e.g. NSAIDs
  – Drugs increasing ciclosporin plasma levels, e.g. ketoconazole and calcium antagonists.

Thus, ciclosporin, in the vast majority of patients, leads to dramatic and early improvement in both clinical and quality of life aspects of psoriasis, especially in the more inflammatory forms. Only in rare cases should ciclosporin treatment be cautiously continued for periods greater than 12–16 weeks in patients with abnormal liver function tests or hypertension, or in elderly individuals. Caution also needs to be entertained when combining ciclosporin with therapies such as phototherapy, particularly PUVA, due to the significantly increased risk of squamous cell carcinoma with long-term therapy.

Systemic retinoids

Systemic retinoids (derivatives of vitamin A) have been utilized in psoriasis therapy for over 25 years. Currently, acitretin is the most commonly prescribed systemic retinoid for psoriasis worldwide. Systemic retinoids modulate epidermal cell proliferation[43], as well as having anti-inflammatory effects.

While acitretin has less efficacy than both methotrexate and ciclosporin, its relative safety profile (see below), excluding teratogenicity, allows for long-term maintenance therapy in a significant proportion of patients, either as monotherapy or in combination with other modalities, particularly phototherapy, which leads to a significant increase in efficacy.

Acitretin as monotherapy leads to slow, gradual, and modest improvement in psoriasis symptomatology when used at the standard dose of 25 mg per day. Unfortunately, higher, more effective doses of acitretin (>40 mg/day) are commonly associated with a significant increase in mucocutaneous side-effects (**291**). In combination with narrowband UVB or PUVA therapy, the dose may be reduced to even 10 mg per day, with significant reduction in side-effects, particularly mucocutaneous, and maintenance of clinical response.

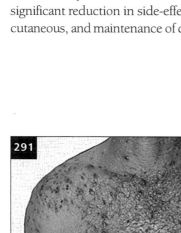

291 Traditional agents. Retinoid side-effects of irritation and scaling in and around lesions.

Side-effects of systemic retinoids
- Mucocutaneous.
- Triglyceride increase.
- Hepatotoxicity infrequent.
- Hair loss in females likely.
- Teratogenicity.

As stated above, acitretin as monotherapy shows only modest efficacy in standard chronic plaque psoriasis; however, in more inflammatory forms, e.g. erythrodermic psoriasis, it shows significantly greater efficacy. This also appears to be the case in patients with palmoplantar disease, particularly the severe hyperkeratotic variety where early desquamation and thinning is noted, even with low-dose 10–25 mg per day. Combination with PUVA and/or narrowband therapy allows for lower dosages of systemic retinoids, and it is also likely that the potential for skin cancers with PUVA therapy are significantly reduced[44]. In addition to combination phototherapy, retinoids in low dosages are often employed to improve response in patients on other forms of systemic therapy, including ciclosporin and biologic agents.

Retinoids and combination therapy

Combination therapy with systemic medications including:
- Sulfasalazine.
- Hydrea.
- Methotrexate (possible increased risk of hepatotoxicity).
- Ciclosporin.
- Azathioprine.
- Biologics.

Combination therapy with UVB and PUVA has the following benefits:
- Superior clinical response.
- Synergistic.
- Decreased acitretin dosage.
- Accelerated response rate.
- Lower UVB/PUVA exposure.
- Shorter treatment periods.
- Decreased total exposure for clearing.

Side-effect profile

Major fetal abnormalities are likely in females exposed to acitretin[45], leading to a 3-year post-acitretin therapy hiatus before conception can be considered (2 years in Europe, 3 years in the United States). The majority of patients on acitretin therapy develop significant muco-cutaneous side-effects, including dry eyes, dry lips, and thinning of the hair[46], particularly in females when higher dosages, i.e. 25–50 mg/day, are utilized. Abnormal liver function tests are seen in a minority of patients, with a significantly lower incidence than with methotrexate therapy; fortunately, however, this is usually completely reversible, with very rare cases of liver fibrosis or cirrhosis being noted (compared to methotrexate). A significant proportion of patients may develop abnormalities in lipid profiles, particularly hypertriglyceridemia. Thus, regular monitoring of liver function studies and lipids is essential, particularly triglyceride levels[45].

Fumaric acid esters

This interesting drug, most commonly used in Germany (since 1995) in a combination of dimethylfumarate and monoethylfumarate, likely functions by inhibiting epidermal cell hyperproliferation, as well as activated T cells[47]. Patients are normally dosed with a combination medication containing 30 mg of dimethylfumarate and 75 mg of monoethylfumarate in an initial one or two tablets a day dosage schedule. Dosage is increased slowly to a maximum of six tablets a day of the full strength combination (120 mg dimethylfumarate and 95 mg monoethylfumarate) in divided dosages twice daily[48,49]. A review of fumaric acid esters has shown a significant improvement in psoriasis after 3 months of therapy when used as monotherapy, or in combination with topical agents[49,50].

Side-effects

The most significant side-effects relating to fumaric acid ester therapy are gastrointestinal issues, with diarrhea, nausea, stomach cramps, and flatulence affecting a significant proportion of patients[47,48]. In addition, flushing may also be seen in up to one third of patients, though it has been observed that this side-effect appears to slowly reduce with continued use of the medication. Other less frequent side-effects include renal and hematologic toxicity, and, rarely, liver toxicity. Thus, patients should be monitored with liver and renal function tests, complete blood counts, with avoidance of other hepatotoxic agents, particularly retinoids and methotrexate.

Second-tier drugs

With the advent of the new biologic agents, the use of medications such as hydroxyurea, 6-thioguanine, and mycophenolate mofetil, previously employed for patients unresponsive to, or with contraindications to traditional agents mentioned above, such as methotrexate, ciclosporin, and retinoids, has been significantly reduced. However, a combination of low-dose acitretin, i.e. 10–25 mg/day with low-dose hydroxyurea (500 mg once or twice daily) has, in our clinic, shown significant effect in maintenance treatment for patients with the hyperkeratotic form of palmoplantar psoriasis.

4 BIOLOGICS

Biologic response modifiers ('biologics,' 'biologicals') are defined by the US Department of Health and Human Services as a 'generic term for hormones, neuro-active compounds, and immunoreactive compounds that act at the cellular level' or as those products 'derived from living material – human, plant, animal, or micro-organism – and used for the treatment, prevention, or cure of disease in humans'[51]. Certainly there is an 'immunologic basis for the treatment of psoriasis with new biologic agents'[52]. Thus, each of the key steps in immunological activation in psoriasis 'offers an opportunity for intervention with engineered biologic therapeutics'[52], thereby blocking molecular activation in individual pathways. The five currently available biologic agents are examples of chimeric antibodies, humanized antibodies, human antibodies, and fusion proteins.

In an excellent review of the value of biologic therapies for psoriasis management[53], it was felt there was a definitive role for these agents due to the 'need for long-term treatment of a chronic disease with potentially safer drugs' than were currently available. Traditional agents are effective in the majority of cases in controlling symptoms for the short term, but have not been documented to be safe with continuous long-term therapy. Likewise, drugs are needed that will be appropriate for all ages and sexes, and not contraindicated in females of childbearing potential. In addition, the article stressed the importance of measuring both physical manifestations and psychosocial issues inherent in psoriasis, an area where the biologic agents have taken the lead in recent years in clinical trials. Finally, in relation to safety, it is important to note that the biological agents, in the main, have fewer organ toxicities than do traditional agents, e.g. hepatotoxicity with methotrexate, nephrotoxicity with ciclosporin, and teratogenicity and mucocutaneous toxicity with systemic retinoids.

A major benefit of biological therapies, particularly the three TNF-α-inhibitory agents discussed below, is the history of their long-term use in diseases as diverse as rheumatoid arthritis, Crohn's disease, ulcerative colitis, and ankylosing spondylitis, both in adults and pediatric patients. To date, over 1,500,000 patients have been treated, many continuously for over 5 years, thus providing an excellent safety database on which to judge the use of these drugs in psoriasis therapy.

Psoriasis is a T-cell-mediated disease. After exposure of the antigen-presenting cell (APC) within the epidermis to an appropriate antigen, cytokines are released, with migration via afferent lymphatics to regional lymph nodes. Thereafter, CD45RO+ T cells migrate back to the skin, where they are activated with the release of multiple cytokines, particularly TNF-α. Thus, even prior to clinically evident skin involvement, T lymphocytes show infiltration into clinically uninvolved skin. The activation of T cells occurs due to interaction between a number of co-stimulatory molecule receptors on T cells and the adjacent APCs[54]. By introducing appropriate T-cell-specific biological agents which target these co-stimulatory molecules, psoriasis patients can be treated more specifically and with less general immune suppression. In addition, as TNF-α is the most significant cytokine increased in psoriatic lesional skin, as well as in joints and nonlesional skin, attempting to reduce circulating TNF-α is a logical step for biological therapy. TNF-α is also an inducible product of keratinocytes and, thus, is a logical target for biological therapy in patients with moderate-to-severe psoriasis, with or without associated psoriatic joint disease.

In this section, we will review relevant data, i.e. clinical efficacy and side-effect profiles of biologic agents currently approved for moderate-to-severe psoriasis (*Table 21*).

T-cell agents
ALEFACEPT
Alefacept is a recombinant fusion protein (human LFA-3-IgG1) designed to prevent interaction between LFA-3 and CD2. Thus, alefacept binds to the CD2 receptor on T lymphocytes, blocking the interaction of LFA-3 and CD2, reducing the activation of T lymphocytes and, hence, the inflammatory component of psoriasis. An important secondary effect of alefacept is programmed cell death (apoptosis) of activated T cells. Alefacept was the first biological agent approved for the treatment of moderate-to-severe psoriasis, in January 2003, in the United States. Initially given as an intravenous 7.5 mg/kg per week injection, the use of alefacept has subsequently been refined to a standard 15 mg I.M. injection given on a weekly basis, for a total of 12 doses. In the initial pivotal study of alefacept, there was a significantly greater reduction in the PASI score at 14 weeks, i.e. 2 weeks after completion of the 12-week course, in the alefacept groups versus placebo. In addition,

Agent	Category	Mode of action	Dosage schedule
ADALIMUMAB	TNF-α inhibitor	Fully human monoclonal IgG1 antibody	80 mg subcutaneous injection at weeks 0 and 1
		Binds to and neutralizes TNF	
		Blocks TNF interaction with p55 and p75 cell-surface TNF receptors	40 mg every other week
		Modulates biological responses induced or regulated by TNF	
ALEFACEPT	T-cell modulator	Recombinant fusion protein (human LFA-3-IgG1)	15 mg intramuscular injection given weekly for a total of 12 weekly dosages
		Binds to CD2 receptor on T lymphocytes, blocking the interaction of LFA-3 and CD2, reducing the activation of T lymphocytes and, hence, the inflammatory component of psoriasis	Minimum 12-week intervals between courses
		Apoptosis of activated T cells	
*EFALIZUMAB	T-cell modulator	Anti-CD11a (hu1124), humanized IgG1 version of the murine anti-human CD11a monoclonal antibody MHM24	1 mg/kg weekly subcutaneous injection
ETANERCEPT	TNF-α inhibitor	Soluble TNF-α receptor	USA: 50 mg twice weekly for 12 weeks; thereafter, 50 mg once weekly
		Prevents TNF-α-mediated cellular response	
		Inhibits interaction of TNF-α with cell-surface receptors	Europe: 50 mg weekly for 24 weeks
INFLIXIMAB	TNF-α inhibitor	Chimeric anti-TNF-α monoclonal antibody human IgG1 constant region joined to a murine-derived antigen-binding variable region	5 mg/kg intravenous infusions at weeks 0, 2, and 6
		Binds with high affinity to both soluble and transmembrane-bound forms of TNF-α	5 mg/kg every 8 weeks thereafter
		Inhibits ability of TNF-α to bind with its receptor, preventing the initiation of intracellular signaling that leads to gene transcription and subsequent biologic activity	
		Produces lysis of TNF-α-producing cells by means of a complement- or antibody-dependent cell cytotoxicity mechanism	
USTEKINUMAB	IL-12/23 inhibitor	Human monoclonal antibody	45 mg for patients weighing <100 kg
		Selectively targets the cytokines interleukin-12 and interleukin-23 (p40 subunit common to both IL-12 and IL-23)	90 mg for patients weighing >100 kg
			Injections given at weeks 0 and 4, then every 12 weeks

*Efalizumab was withdrawn worldwide in early 2009 for use in psoriasis due to three cases of progressive multifocal leukoencephalopathy (PML).

Table 21 **Biologics**. Mode of action and dosage schedule of biologic agents currently approved or in the approval process.

12 weeks post-therapy, a small percentage of patients who had received alefacept alone were almost completely clear of psoriasis. A subsequent phase 3 placebo-controlled clinical trial of intramuscular alefacept in 507 patients with moderate-to-severe psoriasis revealed a PASI 75% reduction with alefacept of 21% versus 5% with placebo after one 12-week course of therapy. Of interest, of the patients in the 15 mg-per-week group who achieved at least 75% PASI reduction 2 weeks after the final dose, 71% maintained at least 50% improvement in PASI throughout the 12-week follow-up period[55].

In both the aforementioned studies, the adverse event profiles were similar in placebo and the treatment groups, with injection site inflammation being classified as mild and restricted to only an occasional patient. There was a slightly higher incidence in infection-related events in the alefacept group than the placebo group, particularly common colds. In each of the two studies, CD4+ cell counts were measured on a weekly basis. There was a trend in the initial study for psoriasis improvement to be correlated with a reduction in CD4 count, although this has not been substantiated in subsequent clinical use. However, the reduction in CD4 counts in the vast majority of patients was not at a level, i.e. <250 cells/mm^3, that is the cut-off point for discontinuation of alefacept therapy. From a safety perspective, CD4 counts are monitored on an every-other-week basis during the 12-week treatment phase, with discontinuation of the weekly alefacept dose until the level has risen above the 250 cells/mm^3 mark.

Efficacy of alefacept[56]

In a recent review of our personal clinical data of 200 patients treated over a 3-year period with alefacept, a small proportion, i.e. 17%, have obtained greater than 6 months remission after a course/courses of alefacept therapy[57]. Patients with stable moderate-to-severe psoriasis, without psoriatic joint disease, and those who have received maximum dosages of methotrexate, ciclosporin, systemic retinoids, or PUVA, are candidates for transition to alefacept, with a gradual 6 to 12-week overlap period as the prior systemic agent is slowly reduced, either at initiation of alefacept therapy or 4 weeks before. The major goal is maintenance of clinical efficacy and, hence, quality of life, without relapse or rebound of psoriasis. With its excellent safety profile, it

would be valuable if a pharmacokinetic or biologic marker could be established for alefacept, as only a minority of patients obtain an excellent response or a subsequent remission with the first course of therapy. A recent study evaluated patients who did not show an adequate response during the first course of therapy, defined as <PASI 50% improvement. With a second course of therapy, 53% of these patients did achieve a PASI 50 response, with incremental efficacy noted over multiple successive 12-week courses of treatment with intervening periods of 12 weeks 'off' therapy[56].

EFALIZUMAB

Efalizumab was the second biological agent approved (November 2003) in the USA and subsequently worldwide for the treatment of moderate-to-severe psoriasis. Efalizumab, or anti-CD11a (hu1124), is a humanized IgG1 version of the murine anti-human CD11a monoclonal antibody MHM24 which recognized human and chimpanzee CD11a[58]. This antibody blocks T-cell-dependent functions mediated by leukocyte function-associated antigen-1 (LFA-1) – an adhesion molecule of central importance in T-cell-mediated responses – including the mixed lymphocyte response (MLR) to heterologous lymphocytes and adhesion of human T cells to keratinocytes. As a result, diapedesis of activated T cells from the circulation into lesional skin is markedly reduced[58].

Clinical efficacy

In a large, multinational study of 793 patients, 529 received 12 weekly dosages of efalizumab versus 264 patients on placebo. In this study, 29.5% of patients achieved PASI 75 versus 2.7% in the placebo arm at the end of the 12-week period. In an interesting long-term study on 290 patients treated for 27 months continuously with weekly efalizumab injections, approximately 50% of patients achieved at least a 75% reduction in PASI score at the end of the 27-month period, with 33% of patients achieving PASI 90 at 18 months[59]. It should be noted that this was an open-label study with the concomitant use of high-potency topical corticosteroids, with phototherapy allowed.

At first, efalizumab showed significant promise in the treatment of plaque psoriasis. In clinical usage, it was found to be particularly effective for the palmoplantar form of psoriasis (**292, 293**).

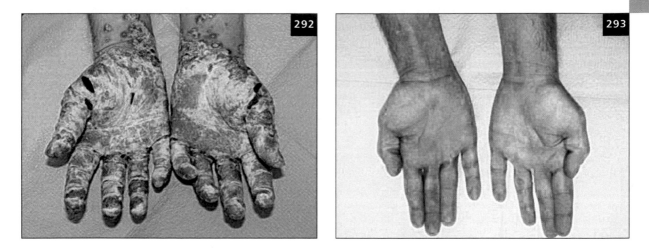

292, 293 **Efalizumab treatment.** Pre- and post-16 weeks efalizumab treatment for palmar psoriasis.

Safety considerations

Efalizumab showed few side-effects in its first 5 years of usage, apart from a small percentage of cases who developed a flare of their disease post-discontinuation of the drug or even in the first 6–10 weeks[60]. However, the finding at the end of 2008 of three cases of progressive multifocal leukoencephalopathy (PML) in patients on long-term efalizumab therapy led to its withdrawal worldwide.

TNF-alpha inhibitory agents

The crucial role of tumor necrosis factor alpha (TNF-α) in the pathogenesis of psoriasis has led to the development of three specific agents currently approved internationally for psoriasis and psoriatic joint disease: etanercept, adalimumab, and infliximab. All three are used individually or in combination with traditional systemic agents – primarily methotrexate – in other disease processes in which TNF-α plays a significant role, including rheumatoid arthritis, Crohn's disease, ulcerative colitis, and ankylosing spondylitis.

ETANERCEPT

Etanercept is a soluble TNF-α receptor that prevents TNF-α-mediated cellular responses by inhibiting the interaction of TNF-α with its cell-surface receptors. Etanercept was first reported in 2000 to be effective in the treatment of 60 patients with psoriatic arthritis and psoriasis[61]. Subsequently, a 24-week double-blind study of etanercept in three separate dosage schedules, i.e. low dose 25 mg once weekly, medium dose 25 mg twice weekly, or high dose 50 mg twice weekly versus placebo over 12 weeks, was evaluated[62]. Results showed a PASI 75% response in 49% of patients in the high-dose group, 34% in the medium-dose group, 14% in the low-dose group, and 4% in the placebo group after 12 weeks of therapy. After 24 weeks, the results for the three dosages of etanercept were 59% PASI 75 in the high-dose group, 44% in the medium-dose group, and 25% in the low-dose group. Etanercept has now been approved in the United States for the treatment of moderate-to-severe psoriasis, with an initial dose of 50 mg twice weekly for 12 weeks, thereafter 50 mg once weekly. In Europe, etanercept is approved in a dose of 50 mg weekly for up to 24 weeks of treatment. In a pivotal study, the psychological and emotional benefits of treatment with etanercept, together with its effect on clinical symptoms of fatigue, were evaluated in 618 patients receiving etanercept 50 mg twice weekly versus placebo, using three separate scoring systems[63]. A meaningful improvement with all three scoring systems was noted versus placebo. Improvements in the fatigue score were correlated with decreasing joint pains, whereas improvements in symptoms of depression in the other two indices were less correlated with objective measures of skin clearance or joint pain. A similar review

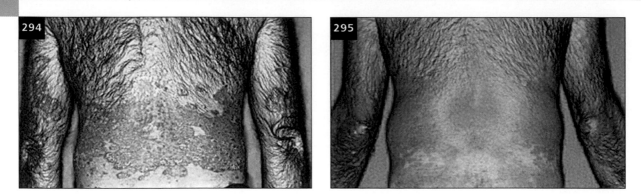

294–295 Etanercept treatment. Pre- and post-24 weeks etanercept.

of the DLQI was evaluated in a multinational random-ized phase III trial of etanercept 50 mg weekly or etaner-cept 50 mg twice weekly versus placebo during an initial 12-week period of treatment. As well as the DLQI, the Short Form-36 survey (SF-36) and patient rating of pru-ritus were evaluated[64]. A significant improvement in all these parameters was noted, thus again confirming the improvement in quality of life in patients on systemic biologic therapy.

As with the other two TNF-α agents, etanercept has a significant effect on the signs and symptoms of psoriat-ic arthritis, with an approximate 55–60% of patients achieving the American College of Rheumatology (ACR) 20% improvement criteria for joint response. Of even greater significance was the inhibition of further radio-graphic joint progression in the etanercept-treated patients at the end of 12 months of treatment[65].

A recent study[66] in 211 patients aged 4–17 years with moderate-to-severe psoriasis, showed that 57% of patients achieved PASI 75 compared to 11% patients on placebo, with no new safety signals noted in this age group, although three episodes of infection occurred, which all resolved without sequelae (**294, 295**).

ADALIMUMAB

Adalimumab is a fully human monoclonal IgG1 anti-body. It binds to TNF and neutralizes the cytokine by blocking its interaction with the p55 and p75 cell-surface TNF receptors, as well as modulating biological responses induced or regulated by TNF[67].

In an initial phase II study utilizing adalimumab in two separate dosages, i.e. 40 mg every other week or 40 mg weekly versus placebo for 12 weeks of blinded therapy, patients were eligible to continue their assigned dosages in a 48-week extension trial, with placebo patients switching to adalimumab 40 mg every other week after 12 weeks[67]. In this study, 53% of patients taking adalimumab every other week, 80% of patients taking adalimumab weekly, and 4% of patients taking placebo achieved PASI 75 response at the end of the 12-week period. These responses were sustained for up to 60 weeks. In a recently completed pivotal, 52-week ran-domized phase III study in adult patients with moder-ate-to-severe psoriasis, adalimumab was studied in 1,212 patients, 814 received adalimumab and 398 placebo, using a dosage schedule of 40 mg adalimumab on an every-other-week basis after a 'loading' dose of 80 mg followed by 40 mg 1 week later. Treatment with adal-imumab was associated with statistically significant improvement in psoriasis, with 71% of adalimumab-treated patients achieving a PASI 75 compared with 7% of placebo-treated patients at week 16[68]. This PASI response was sustained with continuous adalimumab treatment every other week from weeks 16 to 33. Con-tinuation of adalimumab therapy versus placebo from weeks 33 to 52 was associated with a loss of response in 28.4% of patients re-randomized to placebo versus only 4.3% of patients maintained on adalimumab for the ensuing 20 weeks of treatment. Like etanercept, adali-mumab is associated with excellent early response in the treatment of psoriatic joint disease, with similar ACR 20 results noted with the 40 mg every-other-week therapy. In addition, the first randomly controlled trial of a biologic drug versus a traditional systemic agent has recently been completed, namely adalimumab efficacy and safety compared with methotrexate and placebo in patients with moderate-to-severe psoriasis treated over a 16-week period in a multicenter randomized controlled trial. The dosage schedule utilized was adalimumab in a standard dose of 80 mg at week 0 (two 40-mg injections) and thereafter 40 mg every other week until week 16 versus methotrexate in an initial dosing schedule of 7.5 mg at weeks 0 and 1, 10 mg at weeks 2 and 3, and thereafter up to 15 mg or even higher weekly from weeks 4 to 16. After week 8, if PASI 50 was reached, the methotrexate dose could not be increased further. The primary endpoint of the study was a PASI 75 response. At the end of the 16-week period of treatment, 80% of the adalimumab-treated patients achieved PASI 75 versus 36% for methotrexate and 19% for placebo. The response with adalimumab was rapid with a mean percentage PASI improvement noted of 57% at week 4 of treatment.

Adalimumab, like the other two TNF-inhibiting agents, gives 55–60% ACR 20 responses in the treatment of psoriatic arthritis, as well as preventing further radiologic joint destruction.

INFLIXIMAB

Infliximab is a chimeric anti-TNF-α monoclonal antibody, produced by joining the human IgG1 constant region to a murine-derived antigen-binding variable region. Infliximab binds with high affinity to both soluble and transmembrane-bound forms of TNF-α, thus inhibiting the ability of TNF-α to bind with its receptor, preventing the initiation of intracellular signaling that leads to gene transcription and subsequent biologic activity[69].

Multiple randomized controlled studies have been conducted evaluating improvement in psoriasis with infliximab. In two pivotal phase III studies, excellent responses over the course of one year with infliximab were noted[70,71]. In the first trial, 80% of 378 patients treated with infliximab 5 mg/kg at weeks 0, 2, and 6 achieved a PASI 75% response at week 10. At the end of the first year of treatment, 61% of patients in the infliximab-treated arm, infused every 8 weeks, had achieved PASI 75, and an impressive 45% had achieved PASI 90, which, in clinical practice, means almost total clearance of psoriasis. In the second study, 835 patients were randomized to induction therapy with infliximab in two separate dosages, i.e. 3 or 5 mg/kg at the standard weeks 0, 2, and 6 versus placebo. Thereafter, infliximab-treated patients were randomized at week 14 to either traditional, continuous, every-8-weeks dosing or intermittent maintenance regimens based on loss of clinical response. It was shown that the optimal treatment schedule is 5 mg/kg at the standard weeks 0, 2, and 6, and every 8 weeks thereafter. At week 10, 75.5% of patients in the 5-mg/kg infliximab arm achieved PASI 75. At week 50, of all patients randomized at week 14, PASI 75 was achieved by 54.5% of patients in the 5 mg/kg every 8-week arm, with 34.3% of patients achieving a PASI 90 response in the 5 mg/kg arm.

As with etanercept and adalimumab, infliximab also produces a substantial improvement in HRQOL as measured by the DLQI. After three induction infusions at weeks 0, 2, and 6, 40% of patients in the 5-mg/kg infliximab group in a 249-patient double-blind, placebo-controlled trial had achieved a DLQI score of 0, versus 2% of the placebo group, with a strong correlation noted between the PASI response and the DLQI response[72].

As regards psoriatic joint disease, utilizing the standard ACR 20 response at week 14, of 200 patients in an infliximab-versus-placebo double-blind trial, 58% of infliximab-treated patients versus 11% of placebo-treated patients achieved an ACR 20 response, i.e. very similar figures to those achieved by etanercept and adalimumab[73].

Summary

The three TNF-α agents discussed above all show significant responses in the treatment of patients with moderate-to-severe psoriasis, with significant improvement in quality-of-life issues, as well as in psoriatic arthritis. With all three agents there appears to be loss of efficacy in a minority of patients over the course of therapy, as is also seen in rheumatoid arthritis patients. This may necessitate switching from one agent to another, or potentially adjusting the dose where feasible, although cost considerations may militate against this. In addition, in many centers, low-dose methotrexate is utilized in conjunction with TNF-α agent therapy, either *ab initio* as is frequently done with rheumatoid arthritis or at the first sign of loss of clinical efficacy of individual agents. While standard procedure in rheumatology, no meaningful clinical trial data are available for this combination in the treatment of psoriasis, as psoriasis clinical trials of all the biologic agents are, to date, purely monotherapy. Thus, in initiating systemic therapy for psoriasis, it is critical for health care professionals to evaluate, not only the clinical perspective and quality of life perspective, but also for the presence or absence of psoriatic arthritis. Should evident psoriatic arthritis be noted, then, in addition to low-dose methotrexate, initiation of TNF-α therapy has to be strongly considered. The benefit of all three agents in preventing further joint destruction makes for a compelling argument for initiating TNF-α therapy in psoriatic arthritis earlier rather than later (**296, 297**).

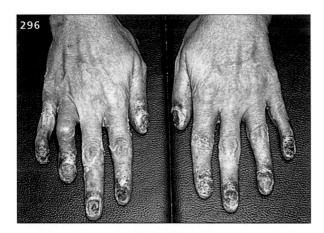

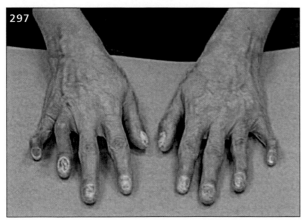

296, 297 Infliximab treatment. Pre- and post-1 year infliximab treatment for the severe acropustulosis form of psoriasis.

Side-effects of TNF-α-inhibiting agents

These are grouped into five major categories:

- **Cardiac failure.** Patients with a history of moderate-to-severe cardiac failure must be evaluated carefully prior to initiation of therapy and especially with infliximab therapy prior to each infusion.
- **Infections.** Both acute infections and granulomatous infections, such as tuberculosis (TB) and histoplasmosis, may be increased in patients undergoing TNF-α-inhibiting therapy (**Tables 22** and **23**). Therefore it is essential to screen for infections at each clinic visit and to evaluate for TB on a yearly basis.
- **Lymphoma**. It is possible that psoriasis patients, like rheumatoid arthritis patients, have an increased baseline lymphoma rate. Whether this is increased further with the use of TNF-α-inhibiting therapy remains to be proven (**Table 24**).
- **Demyelinating neurologic disease.** All patients undergoing TNF-α-inhibiting therapy must be screened for demyelinating conditions, such as multiple sclerosis and optic neuritis, prior to, and at intervals during, therapy. Patients with a history of multiple sclerosis are excluded from therapy (**Table 25**). Care must be taken with patients with a family history of demyelinating neurological disease.
- **Hepatic toxicity**. A small percentage of patients receiving infliximab, e.g. 5% in the clinical studies, were noted to have significant liver enzyme increases. Thus, in addition to periodic monitoring of liver transaminases, careful screening for hepatitis B infection must be undertaken in all patients undergoing TNF-α therapy, at baseline and on a yearly basis. TNF inhibition may, however, be safe for patients with hepatitis C infection.

Finally, because of the infusion delivery of infliximab, appropriate monitoring is important prior to, during, and post-infusion. Experienced nursing staff fully versed in prevention (e.g. antihistamines and acetaminophen) and treatment of infusion-related issues, such as sweating, tachycardia, and hypotension, have allowed for the vast majority of patients selected for infliximab therapy to continue infusions without significant side-effects. Fewer than 1% of patients experience serious infusion-related issues, with a small number of patients also developing a delayed, i.e. 24–72 hour, serum sickness-like reaction, which can be managed with appropriate therapy[74].

	Infliximab*	Etanercept*
Patient-years	590,000	230,000
Histoplasmosis	6.27	0.87
Coccidioidomycosis	1.86	0.43
Tuberculosis	50.0	15.65
Atypical mycobacteria	6.27	4.78
Aspergillosis	4.41	3.04
Cryptococcus	1.89	3.04

*Freedom of information to June 2002

Table 22 TNF-α inhibitors and infections.
Post-marketing reports of granulomatous and
opportunistic infections (per 100,000 patient-years).
[Based on Ruderman and Markenson, ACR 2003]

Recommendations

PPD (purified protein derivative) test for all patients
commencing chronic immunosuppressive treatment,
including biologics:

- ≥5 mm induration is a positive result
- Consider Quantiferon Gold assay for tuberculosis

Evaluation for histoplasmosis and coccidioidomycosis in
endemic areas

Refer to infectious disease consultant as needed, if positive
PPD, pending chest X-ray evaluation

**Table 23 TNF-α inhibitors and granulomatous infec-
tions.** Psoriasis recommendations.

RA data

Prospective study of 18,572 RA (rheumatoid arthritis)
patients enrolled in the National Data Bank for Rheumatic
Diseases 1999–2002

SIR* for lymphoma

- Overall SIR for lymphoma = 1.9 [95% CI 1.3–2.7]
- SIR for biologic use = 2.9 [1.7–4.9]
- SIR for methotrexate (MTX) use = 1.7 [0.9–3.2]
- SIR if not receiving MTX or biologics = 1.0 [0.4–2.5]

Psoriasis data

- Also likely to have two-fold increase for lymphoma

*SIR: standard incidence ratio

Table 24 TNF-α inhibitors and lymphoma.
Patients with rheumatoid arthritis show an increased risk of
lymphoma, possibly as a result of anti-TNF-α therapy,
though current data are insufficient to establish a causal
relationship. [Based on Wolfe, F. and Michaud, K. (2004). Lymphoma in
rheumatoid arthritis. Arthritis and Rheumatism 50(6): 1740–1751]

New onset	Sudden changes
Numbness	Vision
Tingling	Unilateral symptoms
Weakness	
Incoordination	

Table 25 Demyelination and anti-TNF-α therapy.
Clinical signs indicative of demyelination.

IL-12/23 inhibitors

As discussed in Chapter 1, interleukin-12 and -23 also promote inflammation in psoriasis. Produced by activated dendritic cells (DCs), interleukin-12 (IL-12) stimulates production of a T_H1 type, pro-inflammatory milieu, characteristic of psoriasis[75]. Among other actions, IL-12 induces expression of cutaneous lymphocyte antigen (CLA) on the surface of circulating T cells, which binds to E-selectin on vascular endothelial cells of the dermis, and leads to the influx of lymphocytes into the affected skin[76,77]. Indeed, scientists have demonstrated increased levels of IL-12 in psoriatic skin[78].

Also derived from the DC, interleukin-23 (IL-23) similarly fuels inflammation by inducing differentiation of naive T cells into a unique set of T-helper cells – T_H17 cells. These cells, in turn, secrete the proinflammatory cytokines interleukins 17 (IL-17) and 22 (IL-22)[79,80]. Other postulated roles of IL-23 include stimulation of inflammatory mediators inducible nitric oxide synthase (iNOS), interleukin-8 (IL-8), and vascular endothelial growth factor (VEGF)[81], further perpetuating the inflammatory cascade.

A subunit common to both IL-12 and IL-23, IL-12p40, has become the target of extensive drug development. Indeed, a recent large-scale study of genetic association demonstrates increased risk for psoriasis conferred by genes IL-12B and IL-232R, which encode the subunit[82].

USTEKINUMAB

The newest addition to the biologic armamentarium, ustekinumab, highlights the importance of the p40 subunit. Recently approved for treatment of psoriasis in Europe, the USA and Canada, this humanized, monoclonal antibody to the p40 subunit has demonstrated impressive efficacy against psoriatic skin disease in phase III clinical trials[83,84]. These multicenter, randomized, double-blind, placebo-controlled trials – known as PHOENIX I and II – enrolled nearly 2,000 patients with moderate-to-severe psoriasis. Subjects received either 45 mg or 90 mg of ustekinumab at weeks 0 and 4, then every 12 weeks thereafter, or placebo. The primary end-point of the trial was the percentage of subjects who demonstrated a 75% decrease in PASI score at 12 weeks (PASI 75). In sum, 66–76% of treated patients achieved this endpoint, compared to only 3% of controls. As early as week 4, a significant improvement was noted in the treatment groups compared to the placebo group. Peak efficacy was realized at between 20 and 24 weeks, with rates of PASI 75 from 75% to 85%, and was maintained well between doses (**298–301**).

Ustekinumab also demonstrates efficacy against psoriatic joint disease[85]. In a randomized, double-blind, placebo-controlled phase II trial, 146 patients with PsA recalcitrant to disease-modifying antirheumatic drugs (DMARDS) – including non-steroidal anti-inflammatory and anti-TNF-α agents – were enrolled. Subjects received either 63 mg or 90 mg of ustekinumab per week for 4 weeks, followed by placebo at weeks 12 and 16 (group 1) or placebo weekly for 4 weeks, followed by ustekinumab at week 12 and 16 (group 2). The primary end-point was 20% improvement in the American College of Rheumatology inflammatory joint criteria (ACR 20) at week 12. By week 24, the proportion of subjects in group 2 achieving ACR 20 was similar to that of group 1 at week 12 – approximately 42%. Phase III trials, involving larger numbers of patients, are ongoing.

Safety considerations

Of concern with any new systemic therapy, the safety of ustekinumab has been examined closely[86]. In phase II and III clinical trials, 2,266 psoriasis patients received the drug, the vast majority of whom were exposed for more than 6 months. There was no difference in serious adverse events or infections between groups receiving drug and those receiving placebo. Rates of all adverse events did not increase with increased duration of exposure nor cumulative dose of drug. The incidence of cutaneous malignancy was equivalent between groups and non-cutaneous malignancy was less frequent among subjects receiving ustekinumab. Longer-term safety data, i.e. 2–5 years, will need to be evaluated in appropriate registries worldwide.

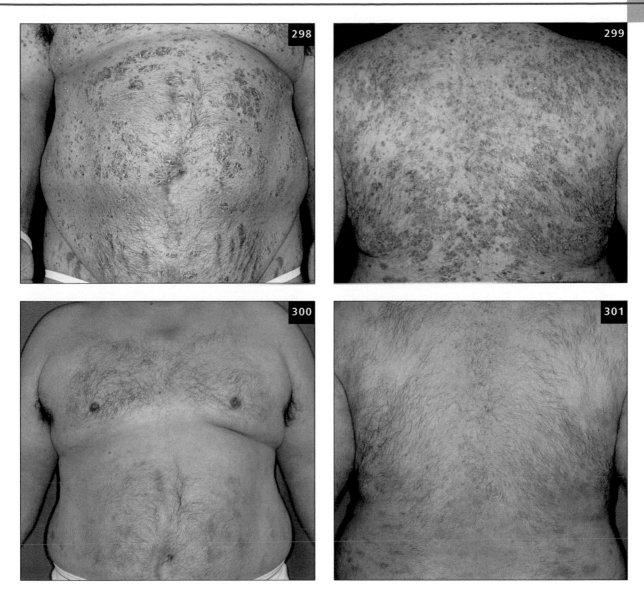

Ustekinumab treatment
298, 299 Pre-therapy.
300, 301 Post-therapy.

COMBINATION, ROTATIONAL, AND SEQUENTIAL REGIMENS

In any chronic disease, where a number of therapeutic options are available, combinations of individual agents are sometimes utilized to reduce the cumulative long-term toxicities from individual treatments while potentially maximizing the duration of remission (*Tables 26, 27*)[87]. In addition, transitioning patients from one systemic agent to another has traditionally been used, especially in the pre-biologic era, to lessen the side-effect potential of the individual systemic agent (*Table 28*).

Historically, combinations of topical agents, phototherapy regimens, and systemic medications have been utilized. The Goeckerman regimen, as discussed previously, was established in the 1920s, using a combination of tar and UVB therapy on an inpatient basis 24 hours per day 7 days per week. Subsequently, this was shortened to a day-care regimen and variations today are still utilized, predominantly as outpatient regimens, where various derivatives of tar are applied in combination with frequent phototherapy. Ingram, in the 1950s,

Factors in considering switch to combination therapy
Monotherapy is not or no longer effective
Cumulative and/or acute toxicity is projected to be less
Side-effects are projected to be fewer
Improved therapeutic outcome (e.g. time, likelihood of clearing)
Increased possibility of tailoring therapy to individual needs

Factors in choosing a particular combination of agents
Severity of disease
Patients' expectations and ease of use
History, relative to use of agents in the combination
Response
Side-effects
Reported efficacy and cost

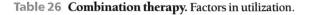

Table 26 Combination therapy. Factors in utilization.

used a combination of anthralin (dithranol), again with UVB phototherapy, to maximize the benefit of each individual agent[10].

Topical combinations

Topical steroids, the mainstay of topical therapy for psoriasis, are also combined with a host of other topical medications including all the vitamin D_3 agents, as well as vitamin A derivatives (tazarotene), in addition to supplementing all forms of phototherapy and systemic therapy. Frequently, the more severe the psoriasis, the more likely for one individual agent to be utilized as the mainstay of treatment, with secondary agents as applicable, i.e. a systemic agent with the use of topical agents for resistant sites such as the scalp and flexural areas.

Topical	Anthralin
	Tar
	Vitamin D_3 analogs
	Vitamin D_3 + topical steroid
	Retinoids
Light treatment	BB-UVB (broadband)
	NB-UVB (narrowband)
	PUVA
Systemics	Ciclosporin
	Fumaric acid esters
	Hydroxyurea
	Methotrexate
	Mycophenolate mofetil (MMP)
	Retinoids
	Sulfasalazine
	Thioguanine
Biological agents	Adalimumab
	Alefacept
	Efalizumab*
	Etanercept
	Infliximab
	Ustekinumab

*withdrawn 2009

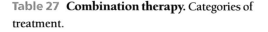

Table 27 Combination therapy. Categories of treatment.

Phototherapy combinations

Both UVB and PUVA are used with topical and systemic agents. Thus, topical tazarotene and calcipotriene enhances both UVB and PUVA therapies[87].

PUVA therapy

The addition of both topical and systemic forms of retinoids has long been used to augment the effect of PUVA therapy. Thus, acitretin combined with PUVA appears to produce a faster clinical response with reduced dosages of the UVA therapy versus therapy with either alone[87–91]. Likewise, systemic retinoids may potentially reduce the carcinogenic effect of long-standing PUVA therapy. In addition to retinoids, other systemic agents are also frequently used with phototherapy, particularly methotrexate, with the one caveat being a rare possibility for a methotrexate-induced 'recall' of ultraviolet light-induced erythema, e.g. prior sunburn[87,92]. While ciclosporin may benefit from augmentation of UVB therapy or PUVA therapy, because of the increased risk of skin cancers inherent with each agent, it is probably wise not to pursue this combination beyond extremely short courses of phototherapy when patients are on maintenance ciclosporin treatment.

Table 28 Combination therapy. Transition/sequential strategies for systemic therapies.

Initial ciclosporin – add acitretin
- Add low-dose acitretin (10–25 mg/day or 25 mg/every other day) to full-dose ciclosporin
- Taper ciclosporin over 3 months
- Gradually increase acitretin according to response
- Monitor lipids carefully
- Maintain on acitretin

Initial acitretin – add ciclosporin
- Both can be given at full dose concurrently
- Acitretin can be tapered or stopped abruptly
- Monitor lipids carefully

Initial methotrexate – add acitretin
- Begin tapering methotrexate over a 2–3 month period
- Introduce acitretin when the patient has been on 7.5 mg/week for 2 months
- Monitor liver enzymes carefully

Initial acitretin – add methotrexate
- Both can be given at full doses concurrently
- Acitretin can be tapered or stopped abruptly
- Monitor liver enzymes carefully

Initial methotrexate – add ciclosporin
- Add low- or full-dose ciclosporin to methotrexate regimen. If previous methotrexate dose is high, reduce dosage immediately (e.g. 30 to ≤20 mg/day)
- Continue ciclosporin until patient responds
- Taper or discontinue ciclosporin following clearing
- Monitor renal function, CBC carefully

Initial ciclosporin – add methotrexate
- Add low-dose methotrexate to ciclosporin regimen
- Continue methotrexate until patient responds
- Taper or discontinue ciclosporin or methotrexate following clearing
- Monitor renal function, CBC carefully

Initial phototherapy – add acitretin
- Decrease phototherapy dose by 50% 1 week after starting acitretin
- Dosimetry may be increased if no phototoxicity occurs
- Add acitretin at 10–25 mg/day
- Gradually increase acitretin until patient has an effective response; 25 mg/day is usually optimal
- Maintain acitretin

Initial acitretin – add phototherapy
- Add phototherapy at 50% usual dose to acitretin regimen
- Acitretin can be tapered or discontinued once clearing occurs

A prior study showed the benefit of combining methotrexate and PUVA, reducing the total cumulative exposure of UVA by approximately 50%, with short courses of methotrexate and PUVA in combination and rotation[93]. Likewise, methotrexate and retinoids have been used in combination for generalized pustular psoriasis[94]. However, caution must be exercised with this approach due to the potential for hepatotoxicity with each individual agent.

Combination of two systemic agents

The combination of ciclosporin and methotrexate has long been utilized by rheumatologists in the treatment of rheumatoid arthritis, especially prior to the introduction of the TNF-α-inhibitory agents[95,96]. Likewise, this combination was relatively commonplace in psoriasis therapy prior to 2003, when the biologic agents became available, with low dosages of each of the two agents being used to minimize individual short-term and long-term toxicities (*Table 29*)[97].

The addition of topical agents to ciclosporin, particularly calcipotriene, has allowed for lower doses of ciclosporin to be effective[98].

Systemic retinoids

Oral retinoids (e.g. acitretin) are considered to be an important combining agent in the treatment of moderate-to-severe psoriasis, having been used with most modalities, particularly ciclosporin[99–107].

Since the development of the biologic agents, all of which are approved as monotherapy for the treatment of moderate-to-severe psoriasis, various traditional systemic agents have been utilized in combination with the biologic agents, especially in order to increase clinical efficacy. While the majority of studies with TNF-α-inhibitory agents for rheumatoid arthritis and Crohn's have been in combination with agents such as methotrexate and low-dose prednisone, all clinical trials in psoriasis with TNF-α agents and T-cell agents, as discussed under Biologics above, have been as monotherapy. Therefore, data utilizing biological agents in combination with traditional agents in psoriasis patients are lacking.

Combination therapy is used to maximize efficacy and minimize toxicity, utilizing agents with different modalities of action, different kinetics, and separate toxicities to achieve these goals. Retinoids may be of particular value in reducing the squamous cell carcinomata, especially in patients with prior PUVA therapy.

Table 29 **Combination therapy.** Therapeutic options using traditional and systemic agents.

Lower dose to achieve response	Sequential therapy to achieve quick response	Rotational therapy to avoid cumulative toxicity
MTX + CyA	MTX + retinoid	MTX → Retinoid → UV
MTX + retinoid	CyA + retinoid	Repeat cycles
UV + retinoid		

Table 30 **Rotational therapy.** Factors in the selection of traditional, non-biologic rotational agents.

Biological agents used in combination therapy[108]
T-CELL AGENTS
Alefacept

In a personal series of 200 patients treated with alefacept over a 3-year period, a number of drugs were successfully combined with alefacept, mainly to increase the initial response to therapy, including methotrexate, systemic retinoids, and short courses of phototherapy. In addition, alefacept has been combined with methotrexate in the treatment of psoriatic arthritis, with added benefit over methotrexate monotherapy[109].

TNF-α-INHIBITING BIOLOGIC AGENTS
Etanercept, infliximab, and adalimumab

As stated previously, a significant number of clinical trials have been performed in rheumatoid arthritis and inflammatory bowel disease, whereby traditional drugs, particularly methotrexate, are used in combination with anti-TNF-α agents. Thus, from our personal experience, if patients appear to be having suboptimal clinical response to one of these three agents, or begin to lose response after a period of time, the addition of low-dose methotrexate, i.e. 7.5–10 mg, is frequently rewarding. This is possibly due, in part, to its effect on reducing or inhibiting antibody production. Likewise, systemic retinoids in low dosages, e.g. acitretin 10 mg daily, as well as phototherapy, is likely to produce a similar benefit.

Rotational therapy

The concept of rotational therapy was originally proposed by Drs Weinstein and White. Four specific therapies, i.e. methotrexate, PUVA, etretinate, and UVB (with or without concomitant tar) were used in a rotational approach, selecting each individual therapy for approximately 12–24 months followed by rotating to one of the other three treatments. Thus, potential morbidity and side-effects are minimized for each individual therapy and long-term clinical remission is maintained, and, hence, quality of life (*Tables 30, 31*)[110].

When to rotate
Onset of new flare
Agent becomes ineffective
Toxicity or intolerable side-effects with current agents
At a set time (e.g. 12–24 months)
When cumulative dose approaches toxicity

Choice of next agent
Desired outcome by patient
Past medications and response
Side-effects
Cost

Switch to secondary agents
Cumulative toxicity precluded primary agents
Unacceptable side-effects of primary agents
Primary agents ineffective

Frequency of rotation	
Response	
Maintenance	– dose
	– effectiveness of topicals as adjuncts
Side-effects	

Topical + light
Goeckerman, Ingram
Vitamin D_3 + PUVA or UVB
Tazarotene + PUVA or UVB

Systemic + light
Methotrexate + UVB or PUVA
Retinoids + UVB or PUVA

Topical + systemic
All topicals with all systemics

Systemic + systemic
Methotrexate + ciclosporin
Ciclosporin + retinoids
Hydroxyurea + retinoids
Fumaric acid esters + retinoids

Systemic + light + topical
Methotrexate, retinoids, sulfasalazine, others + UVB/PUVA + topicals

Table 31 **Rotational therapy.** Combination and rotational possibilities.

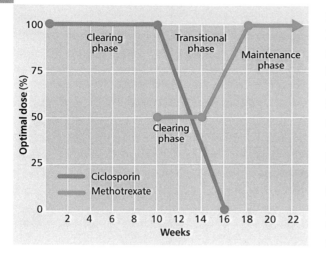

302 Sequential therapy. Maintenance (overlap) therapy with ciclosporin and methotrexate. Ciclosporin can be discontinued after approximately 16 weeks.

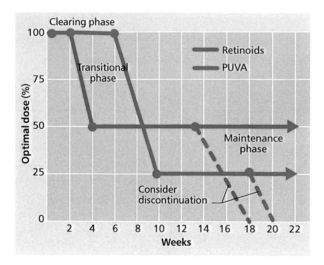

303 Sequential therapy. Retinoids–PUVA approach.

Sequential therapy

Dr John Koo first proposed a strategy designed to optimize initial efficacy, leading to safe maintenance regimens using specific combinations, with a three-step combination schedule in a specific sequence. This involved a clearing phase utilizing a powerful rapidly acting agent, such as ciclosporin (in the prebiologic era), then a transitional phase in which a well-tolerated potentially safer agent, such as acitretin, is introduced with gradual tapering of the initial clearing agent (ciclosporin). Finally came the third phase, the maintenance phase, in which the patient remains on the maintenance drug, with additional therapies to include phototherapy, topical agents, etc., as required (**302, 303**)[87,111].

In summary, with the introduction of biologic agents in 2003, a number of patients who had been maintained beyond the normal period of time on individual traditional agents, such as ciclosporin, methotrexate, and PUVA, now had potentially safer longer-term agents available to them. In order to prevent the usual relapse or even rebound with discontinuation of the traditional agents, a slow tapering approach of the prior agent was used in a sequential fashion, while introducing the newer biologic agent with gradual discontinuation over a period of 4–8 weeks of the prior traditional agent. Pending the response of the introduced biologic agent, this period could be shortened or lengthened accordingly. Should the psoriasis be accompanied by documented psoriatic joint disease, then the need for combination therapy would be enhanced, i.e. a TNF-α-inhibitory agent with low-dose methotrexate or a nonsteroidal anti-inflammatory drug (NSAID). In addition, as with rheumatoid arthritis, a number of rheumatologists would introduce methotrexate–TNF-α-inhibitory agents in combination as the first-line therapy.

Psoriasis patients are thus fortunate in having available to them a wide array of therapeutic agents, including topicals, various wavelengths of light, narrowband UVB and PUVA therapy, together with various forms of traditional systemic agents and the newer biologic agents. While they can all be used as traditional monotherapy, the ability to combine the different classes of agents in order to minimize toxicities and potentially maintain long-term clinical response and, hence, improve quality of life in the psoriasis population, is appealing .

FUTURE DIRECTIONS

The wave of drug development that has led to the biologic revolution in psoriasis shows no signs of slowing (*Table 32*)[112]. As scientists probe deeper into the pathogenesis of inflammation in general and psoriasis specifically, new therapeutic targets emerge. Novel drugs are not the only source of interest, however. In time, researchers hope to confirm the safety profiles of existing newer agents, like the biologics. Furthermore, early trials comparing biologics with one another and with traditional counterparts, such as methotrexate, reveal important data on comparative efficacy. Even laser technology enters the therapeutic arsenal, targeting localized disease. Finally, genetic profiles using microRNA arrays may soon predict the effectiveness and individual risk profiles of medicines in a given population of psoriatics, an emerging field known as pharmacogenomics. Indeed, the future for the skin of psoriasis sufferers seems not only bright but, possibly, clear.

Cytokines

Regulators of cell interaction and activity, cytokines play pivotal roles in the creation and maintenance of inflammation. As such, these small proteins provide a prime target for drug therapy in inflammatory diseases, like psoriasis.

A long-awaited, head-to-head comparison of adalimumab with methotrexate favors the biologic, in terms of efficacy and side-effect profile[113]. The CHAMPION study represents the first phase III, randomized, double-blind, placebo-controlled trial comparing efficacy of 'old standard' methotrexate with a biologic, specifically adalimumab. After 16 weeks of either adalimumab at standard dosing, methotrexate dosed up to 25 mg weekly, or placebo, 79.6% of patients treated with adalimumab achieved PASI 75 compared to only 35.5% and 18.9% of those receiving methotrexate or placebo, respectively. Patients treated with methotrexate experienced the greatest number of adverse events, warranting discontinuation of the study.

Data from the phase III ACCEPT trial, the first to directly compare two biologic agents, demonstrated the superiority of ustekinumab over the time-tested, TNF-α-inhibitory agent etanercept[114]. In this randomized, single-blind, phase III study, 903 patients with moderate-to-severe psoriasis received either ustekinumab (45 mg or 90 mg) at baseline and week 4, or etanercept 50 mg twice-weekly for 12 weeks. The primary end-point, PASI 75 at 12 weeks, was achieved in 67.5–73.8% of the ustekinumab group compared to 56.8% of the etanercept group. An impressive PASI 90 was reached in 36–45% of the ustekinumab group versus 23% of the etanercept group at 12 weeks.

Name	Mechanism of delivery	Mechanism of action	Phase
ABT-874	Injection	IL-12/IL-23 inhibitor	III
AIN 457A2211	Injection	Anti IL-17A antibody	I
AMG-827	Injection	IL-17R	II
BG-12	Oral	Fumaric acid ester	III
CC-10004 (apremilast)	Oral	TNF-alpha inhibitor	II
CP-690,550	Systemic and topical	JAK inhibitor	II
CTAO18	Topical	Vitamin D analog	II
CTAR398	Topical	Vitamin D analog	II
ILV-094	Infusion	IgG1 antibody	I
ISA-247	Oral	Calcineurin inhibitor	III
LY-2439821	Infusion	IL-17A	I

Table 32 **Selected new drugs in development.** Phase I of clinical trials determines the safety of a new drug, phase II assesses its effectiveness, and phase III examines both safety and efficacy in large groups of people.

[Adapted from the National Psoriasis Foundation website: www.psoriasis.org/research/pipeline/chart.php]

Recent data assessing another fully human, anti-IL 12p40 antibody (ABT-874) support the central role of IL-12 and IL-23 in psoriasis pathogenesis[115]. Results from a phase II, randomized, double-blind, placebo-controlled trial of ABT-874 involving 180 patients reveal an impressive 90–93% of those receiving multiple treatments achieved PASI 75 at 12 weeks. Patients tolerated the injectable treatment well, rarely developing minor injection-site reactions and upper respiratory tract infections.

With the recent understanding of the important role of T_H17 cells in the immunopathogenetics of psoriasis (see p.17), antibodies to T_H17 are in early stages of clinical trials. Likewise, antibodies to other key cytokines, especially interleukins, are undergoing evaluation.

Growth factors

For over a decade, scientists have recognized the role of aberrant angiogenesis in the development of psoriasis. A key mediator, VEGF, is increased in psoriatic plaques[116]. Furthermore, serum levels of the vascular growth factor appear to parallel clinical disease severity, and single-nucleotide polymorphisms in the gene encoding VEGF confer risk for early-onset psoriasis[117,118]. Remarkably, delivery of VEGF genes to mice resulted in a psoriasiform phenotype[119]. Equally exciting, the antagonist VEGF Trap reversed the condition in affected mice. A monoclonal antibody to VEGF, bevacizumab, has been approved for a variety of neoplasms, leading scientists to speculate about its application in other disease states including psoriasis[120,121].

Calcineurin inhibitors

Close relatives of traditional agents are also under investigation. The calcineurin inhibitors, a class of drug in which ciclosporin is the eldest member, inhibit T-cell activation by inactivating a key enzyme necessary for stimulating the transcription factor NF-AT (nuclear factor of activated T cell). Without activated NF-AT, genes required for B-cell and further T-cell activation lie dormant and immunity is suppressed. As discussed above, significant nephrotoxicity, hypertension, and malignancy risk limit long-term use of ciclosporin. However, the development of closely related oral pimecrolimus, systemic counterpart to the well-known topical agent, excited researchers with its similar efficacy to ciclosporin, but purportedly lesser effects on renal tubules and blood pressure[122]. Unfortunately, the risk of lymphoproliferative disorders has currently halted development[108].

Another calcineurin inhibitor, ISA-247, has stirred interest in the psoriasis research community. In a phase II trial, 1.5 mg/kg per day of ISA-247 resulted in a PASI 75 in 66% of patients at 12 weeks[123]. The serum creatinine level rose mildly in those treated but remained within normal limits. Whether the rise heralds significant renal toxicity can only be assessed with longer-term follow-up.

Lasers

Heinrich Koebner, who described the development of psoriasis in areas of skin trauma over 100 years ago, might have been amazed at the notion of 'physical' treatments for psoriasis. However, with advances in laser technology, both the excimer and pulsed-dye lasers join the therapeutic armamentarium for limited disease. The excimer laser delivers 308-nm radiation to affected skin with promising results[124]. Side-effects include erythema, blistering, and hyperpigmentation. The pulsed-dye laser may benefit often recalcitrant palmoplantar psoriasis, especially when used in combination with salicylic acid and/or topical calcipotriol[125].

Pharmacogenomics

Decoding of the human genome has launched a brave new world in medicine. Psoriasis researchers have embraced this exciting technique, with hopes of tailoring specific treatment regimens according to an individual's unique genetic, phenotypic, and biochemical profile. The use of biologic markers, such as allelic and protein polymorphisms, to predict response to therapy loosely defines the new and exciting field of pharmacogenomics. Even in its infancy, the field has already been applied to several traditional therapies for psoriasis. Polymorphisms in the metabolic enzyme thymidylate synthetase, for example, may forecast the efficacy and side-effect profile of methotrexate[126]. Furthermore, variations in VEGF may predict response to acitretin via effects on all-trans retinoic acid[127]. Similar studies assessing the newer biologic agents are under way.

6 EFFECTS OF PSORIASIS ON QUALITY OF LIFE

ACCORDING TO A RECENT SURVEY, 79% of patients with severe psoriasis believe the disease negatively affects their lives (304)[1]. Sufferers often fear social gatherings, face discrimination at work, and, with alarming frequency, 'wish [they were] dead'[2–4]. The devastating effects of psoriasis include impairment of physical, psychological, social, and occupational functioning. The psoriasis clinical and research community evaluates these domains scientifically, a process formally known as health-related quality of life (HRQOL) assessment[5]. Striking results have emerged, stressing the importance of evaluating HRQOL, not just body surface area (BSA), when determining the extent of disease and subsequent initiation and alteration of systemic therapy[6].

PHYSICAL IMPAIRMENT

Within the HRQOL assessment, physical impairment encompasses declines in mobility, activities of daily living, energy, and sleep[7]. To the surprise of many, deficits in physical functioning associated with psoriasis rival those of debilitating diseases such as cancer, diabetes, hypertension, and major depressive disorder[8]. By one account, 26% of psoriatics alter their daily activities directly as a result of the disease[4]. Insomnia leads to fatigue and poor job performance[1,4,7]. As many as 59% of patients surveyed report significant time missed from work for treatments[3].

Sadly, patients of lower socioeconomic standing shoulder a greater burden of disease than higher-earning counterparts[9]. A recent survey by the National Psoriasis Foundation found that patients with severe disease (i.e. greater than 10% BSA) were more likely to earn below $30,000 (£20,000) per year. In a separate survey, 42% of psoriatics polled report financial difficulty and concern about being fired[1]. Monetary unease tends to affect men more than women[10]. Likewise, patients in this group appear to do less well on therapy[11].

The presence of psoriatic arthritis (PsA) compounds the physical impairment associated with skin disease. According to a recent survey, 60% of participants with PsA report difficulty walking, standing, or using their hands[1]. Compared to patients with rheumatoid arthritis (RA), patients with PsA experience more bodily pain[10].

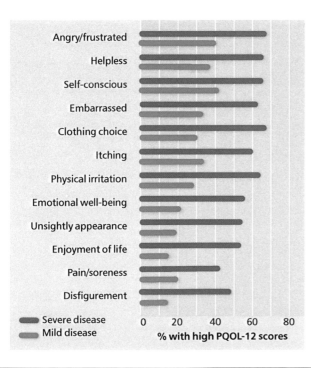

304 Psoriasis and quality of life. A survey of 91 patients with very severe psoriasis and 97 with mild psoriasis showed that even mild disease had a pronounced impact. Patients rated questions (Koo–Menter Psoriasis Instrument, PQOL-12) from 0 to 10, with 8–10 being a high score.

National Psoriasis Foundation Spring Survey Panel 2004.

PSYCHOSOCIAL IMPAIRMENT

Psoriasis affects the mind as well as the body. Disturbing data published in the 1990s revealed that 5.5% of psoriatics surveyed had active suicidal ideation and 9.7% had a death wish[2,12]. Psoriasis patients suffer from low self-esteem, rating themselves as unattractive and sexually undesirable[1,13]. Feelings of embarrassment, helplessness, and frustration prevail, particularly among unmarried patients under 55 years[10,14,15]. Major depressive disorder frequently affects patients with psoriasis (see also p.123), as severity of depression tends to correlate with area of skin involvement and symptoms such as pruritus[12,16–18].

Psoriatics loath social situations involving skin exposure and tend to avoid activities such as swimming in public pools and participating in sporting events[1,19]. Indeed, psoriasis sufferers worry incessantly about how others view their disease, a phenomenon that, in one study, influenced overall quality of life even more than general health status[20]. The disease also affects sexual intimacy, depressing both desire and function[21,22]. In a study from 1997, 49 of 120 psoriatics surveyed (40.8%) reported a decline in sexual activity[22]. This group also suffered greater arthralgia, pruritus, and scaling, as well as depressive symptoms and alcohol abuse.

In some instances, the psoriatics' anxiety about how others perceive them may be warranted. Indeed, disease sufferers experience unequal treatment in a variety of settings, including the workplace. According to a survey from the National Psoriasis Foundation, 6% of those polled recount discrimination on the job as a direct result of their skin disease[1]. Another revealing study found that, among 100 patients with psoriasis, 19% suffered at least 50 episodes of rejection, often occurring at work[23]. Experiences of rejection, in turn, correlated with seeking medical attention and, ironically, impairment of job performance.

Fortunately, certain strategies for coping with psoriasis diminish its effect on HRQOL. Informing others that psoriasis is not contagious, according to one compelling study, was associated with smaller decrements in HRQOL[24]. Conversely, strategies such as covering affected skin and avoiding interaction with others correlated with greater declines. Other effective means of coping, based on a longitudinal study of Dutch psoriatics, include communicating emotions about the disease to others, seeking social support, and attempting to distract oneself from awareness of the disease[25].

ASSESSMENT TOOLS

Awareness that diseases like psoriasis so dramatically alter the lives of those affected represents only one part of the HRQOL assessment. Determining the magnitude of this effect poses another challenge. In response, researchers have produced a myriad of assessment tools designed to quantify the effects of diseases on HRQOL (see Appendix for a range of examples). Some tools apply to all diseases, others only to dermatological conditions, and others still specifically to psoriasis (*Table 33*). Ideally, objective measures of HRQOL provide clinicians with yet another marker of disease severity, important when considering alteration and effectiveness of therapy, for example. These tools also allow for broad comparisons of HRQOL between patients suffering from vastly different diseases.

Generic measures
Short Form 36 (SF-36)

In 1993, researchers introduced SF-36[26–28]. The tool, composed of 36 items, assesses eight general domains: physical functioning, pain, vitality, social functioning, mental health, general health perceptions, and role limitations due to physical and emotional impairment. Despite its broad scope, SF-36 correlates moderately well with PASI[29]. Ironically, SF-36 may even be superior to HRQOL tools specific to dermatology when evaluating patients with certain skin conditions for psychological and physical impairment[30,31]. Such diseases include hand eczema, in which a relatively small area of disease causes great functional and emotional incapacity. Further, SF-36 has been used as an outcome measure in several clinical trials involving PsA[32,33].

Critics of the application of SF-36 to psoriasis point out that physical disability weighs more heavily than psychological[20]. Consequently, the tool may undervalue the embarrassment and isolation experienced by often fully-functioning patients with psoriasis. Within the realm of clinical trials for psoriasis, the tool also reportedly failed to differentiate between treatment and placebo groups[4].

Health Assessment Questionnaire (HAQ)

Originally designed for patients with arthritis, the HAQ measures five broad dimensions, comprising disability, pain and discomfort, adverse treatment effects, monetary cost of treatment, and death[34]. Abridged versions for the spondyloarthropathies (HAQ-S) and psoriasis

Assessment tools		
Generic	Short Form (SF)-36	
	Health Assessment Questionnaire (HAQ)	
Dermatological	Dermatology Life Quality Index (DLQI)	
Psoriasis-specific	Psoriasis Disability Index (PDI)	
	Salford Psoriasis Index (SPI)	
	Koo–Menter Psoriasis Instrument (KMPI)	
Psoriatic arthritis	American College of Rheumatology – 20% responder criteria (ACR-20)	
	Psoriatic Arthritis-specific Quality of Life (PsAQoL) instrument	

Table 33 HRQOL assessment tools.

(HAQ-SK) also exist. Scores on the HAQ and its variants correlate well with physical disability among PsA patients, but not with PASI[35]. Experts conclude that the tools adequately assess physical impairment from joint disease, but fall short in evaluating the psychological and social effects on those with disease limited to the skin[4].

Tools for dermatology
Dermatology Life Quality Index (DLQI)
Archetype among QOL tools for skin disease, the 10-item DLQI is a well-studied instrument that covers a wide range of domains, including symptoms, feelings, daily activities, leisure, work and school, relationships, and treatment[36]. Subjects complete each item by ticking a box next to the most appropriate response on a four-point Likert scale. Total scores range from 0, conveying no QOL impairment, to 30. All items refer to experiences during the preceding week only.

Since its inception in 1994, the tool has been used in nearly 100 research studies, spanning 17 countries, and appears in more than 20 languages[31]. DLQI maintains high internal consistency and reproducibility. Furthermore, the tool has successfully discriminated treatment from placebo groups in many clinical trials and correlates well with an HRQOL index designed specifically for psoriasis, the psoriasis disability index (PDI, see below)[4,37].

Psoriasis-specific
Psoriasis Disability Index (PDI)
For over two decades, psoriasis researchers have measured HRQOL with the PDI. This 15-item tool encompasses daily activities including work and school, personal relationships, leisure and treatment, all over the preceding month[38–40]. A revised edition of the tool allows for two methods of scoring each item: the first a visual scale rated one to seven, the other a four-point scale using tick boxes. In either case, higher scores represent greater disability.

Despite limited validation initially, the PDI has been used in over 30 publications across 20 countries. Over the lifetime of the tool, researchers have compared PDI to other well-established QOL and disease severity measures of psoriasis, demonstrating moderate correlation with PASI and SF-36 and high correlation with DLQI[41–43]. PDI also shows sensitivity to the outcomes of treatment, such as ultraviolet light, for patients with severe psoriasis[44]. Sensitivity diminishes, however, in patients with mild to moderate disease[4].

Salford Psoriasis Index (SPI)
A relative newcomer among HRQOL measures for psoriasis, the SPI assesses three broad aspects of psoriatic disease, including PASI score, psychosocial disability, and historical severity of disease[45]. The former two domains are each converted to a numerical score, 0 to 10. The latter, scored 0 to 5, is based on prior systemic therapies, hospitalizations, and episodes of erythroderma. A result from the index is expressed with three numerical values, each representing one of the domains above. A score of 10:10:5, for example, represents maximal disease severity. Results of the SPI correlate modestly with PASI[45]. The index also demonstrates high sensitivity to treatment-mediated changes in HRQOL[46].

Koo–Menter Psoriasis Instrument (KMPI)
The growing movement to consider HRQOL in management decisions for psoriasis patients resulted in the KMPI. Specifically, the tool incorporates assessments of QOL, BSA, symptoms and signs suggestive of PsA, as well as selected other domains[47]. The creators sought to provide psoriasis caregivers with a tool to guide decisions about the initiation of systemic therapy[48].

The two-page instrument includes a section in which the patient evaluates his or her own disease, in terms of quality of life, location and severity of skin involvement, and symptoms of inflammatory arthritis. The 12 items of the tool appraising quality of life, known as the psoriasis-specific HRQOL 12-item scale (PQOL-12), derive from a 41-item questionnaire that has been extensively validated[49,50]. The patient scores each item of the PQOL-12 from 0 to 10, with higher values representing greater impairment. A total score of 50 or higher corresponds to significant decrement in HRQOL[4].

The KMPI requires only 5 minutes to complete. A recent trial involving the oral retinoid tazarotene demonstrated the tool's sensitivity to changes in disease state, as measured by more traditional means, such as PASI[51]. Despite significant utilization in the United States since its publication in 2003, however, the KMPI remains relatively new to the field with validation against more well-established measures of HRQOL still to be undertaken.

Outcome measures in psoriatic arthritis
American College of Rheumatology – 20% responder criteria (ACR-20)

As the success of drugs is increasingly determined by clinical trials, the American College of Rheumatology sought to standardize the definition of 'adequate response' to treatment with the release of 20% responder criteria (ACR-20, see Appendix) in 1995[52]. Treatment is deemed 'successful' with 20% improvement in the number of both swollen and tender joints, as well as three of five other items (see Appendix). Although not designed solely to assess HRQOL, items concerning functional status and patients' global assessment may reflect this domain. Originally created for clinical trials involving RA, the ACR-20 has since been employed in trials for PsA therapy, including biological agents etanercept, infliximab, and adalimumab[33, 53, 54].

Psoriatic Arthritis-specific Quality of Life instrument (PsAQoL)

Despite the potentially devastating impact of PsA on patients, relatively few assessment tools dedicated to its effects on HRQOL are available[55]. In 2004, clinical researchers in the United Kingdom introduced the 20-item Psoriatic Arthritis-specific Quality of Life instrument (PsAQoL) (see Appendix)[56]. Derived directly from interviews with PsA patients, the tool demonstrated excellent internal consistency and test–retest reliability. Unfortunately, the use of PsAQoL in clinical trials has been limited thus far.

Rheumatoid arthritis as a model for HRQOL assessment

Unfortunately, the psoriasis community lacks a method of systematic evaluation and standardization of the various HRQOL assessment tools described above. Researchers may look to the example set by rheumatologists in response to similar issues surrounding rheumatoid arthritis (RA). A collaborative, data-driven effort known as Outcome Measures in Rheumatoid Arthritis Clinical Trials (OMERACT) seeks to standardize outcome measures in RA[57]. A web-based program, the OMERACT filter, assesses the various QOL tools for validity (face, content, construct, and criterion), fiscal feasibility, and discriminatory ability[58]. The program provides a grade for each outcome measure, permitting and encouraging objective comparison with other tools.

CONCLUSION

Despite problems with standardization, QOL measures in psoriasis maintain strength in number. A disease that devastates in so many ways warrants great nuance in measuring HRQOL. Experts suggest that, for conditions with such far-reaching psychological and physical effects, incorporating several outcome measures may be necessary to adequately capture all aspects of HRQOL[4]. It is hoped that the near future will bring filters analogous to the OMERACT for measures in psoriasis, ensuring the greatest possible validity and more widespread use in clinical practice. Perhaps then the medical community and even the general public will appreciate what psoriasis sufferers understand all too well. To an increasing degree in this disease, severity is in the eyes of the afflicted.

7 PSORIASIS AS A SYSTEMIC DISEASE

PSORIASIS CORRELATES with diseases well beyond the scope of dermatology, challenging its age-old perception as merely 'a malady of the skin.' Indeed, a growing body of work links psoriasis to disorders in a wide range of organ systems, cardiovascular to psychiatric (305). Whether these associations result from a single, systemic disease process, genetic association or a confounding feature, such as toxic therapy or substance abuse, remains to be elucidated with further study of pathophysiology. Nonetheless, with the discovery of each disease association and common pathogenic pathway, the psoriasis paradigm shifts from a disease of a single organ to a systemic condition with the skin but one of several vehicles for expression[1].

CARDIOVASCULAR DISEASE

Myocardial infarction

For decades researchers have recognized the potential connection between psoriasis and myocardial infarction (MI). Early studies, while supportive of the association, were criticized because of small sample sizes, hospital-based design, and failure to control confounding risk factors for coronary artery disease[2–5]. A landmark work from 2006 established the relationship more soundly using population-based data from the United Kingdom collected prospectively[6]. Specifically, researchers utilized a database considered representative of the British population to track a cohort of over 130,000 patients with psoriasis and 556,000 controls for occurrences of MI over 15 years. Investigators stratified the cohort according to severity of skin disease and controlled for established risk factors for MI, including sex, age, diabetes mellitus (DM), hypertension (HTN), hyperlipidemia, smoking, and body mass index (BMI). Striking results emerged as the relative risk of MI, adjusted for risk factors, was higher in each subgroup of patients

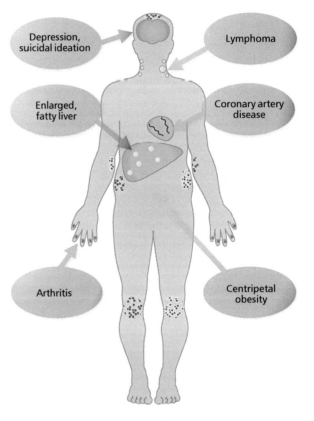

305 Psoriasis as a systemic disease. Psoriasis has been consistently linked to a wide variety of diseases affecting other organs.

with psoriasis compared to controls. Young subjects with severe disease maintained the greatest relative risk[7].

The authors proposed a pathogenic mechanism common to both psoriasis and MI: a dysfunctional immune state in which pro-inflammatory T_H1 cells and cytokines such as TNF-α dominate, a prevailing theory[8]. Investigators cite studies involving patients with rheumatoid arthritis, another T_H1-dependent disease, who also demonstrate higher rates of MI[9,10].

Psoriasis sufferers appear more prone to high-risk behaviors linked to MI as well. Paramount among them, cigarette smoking amplifies risk for MI at least two- to three-fold by a broad array of mechanisms, including hastened progression of atherosclerosis, damage to coronary artery endothelium, enhanced inflammation, and aberrant platelet aggregation[11]. Both hospital- and population-based studies demonstrate a higher prevalence of smoking among psoriatics from the United Kingdom, Germany, Italy, and Utah compared to those without disease, with odds ratios (ORs) ranging from 1.31 to 2.96[12–14].

An extensive review of the potential connections between psoriasis and cardiac disease is available[15]. The authors discuss evidence linking psoriasis to traditional risk factors for coronary artery disease – such as HTN, DM, hyperlipidemia, smoking, and alcohol consumption – discussed below. Intriguing, less conventional risk factors associating heart disease with psoriasis, such as elevated homocysteine levels, are also noted. The authors speculate that chronic inflammation and immune dysregulation likely serve as the common underlying link to both diseases. They further call for longitudinal studies aimed at confirming the risk of heart disease in psoriatics directly.

Features of metabolic syndrome

Definition of the metabolic syndrome requires three or more of the following:

Waist circumference >40 inches (102 cm) in men, >35 inches (89 cm) in women

Blood pressure >135/85 mmHg

HDL cholesterol <40 mg/dl in men, <50 mg/dl in women

Triglycerides >150 mg/dl

Fasting blood sugar >100 mg/dl

Table 34 Metabolic syndrome. This collection of risk factors combines to increase the likelihood of cardiovascular disease.

METABOLIC DISORDERS

The metabolic syndrome

The concurrence of certain metabolic derangements, such as insulin resistance and dyslipidemia, has led scientists to describe a broad state of metabolic disarray characterized by cumulative risk for vascular disease greater than the sum of risk conferred by its individual components[16]. The metabolic syndrome, also known ominously as syndrome X, encompasses abnormalities in blood pressure, lipid metabolism, insulin utilization, and body habitus (**Table 34**)[17]. Staggering data suggest the prevalence of the syndrome to be 7–26% across Europe and 24% in the United States[18–23].

Three large-scale studies assessed the prevalence of the metabolic syndrome, and its constituent components, among patients with psoriasis[12–14]. In a study of hospitalized German patients,[12] investigators compared 581 patients with psoriasis to 1,044 controls, demonstrating an OR of 5.29 for the combined features of metabolic syndrome. Specific elements of the syndrome were more common among psoriasis sufferers, as well, including hypertension (OR = 3.27), diabetes mellitus type II (OR = 2.48), hyperlipidemia (OR = 2.09), and obesity, defined as BMI greater than 30 (OR = 2.3).

A similar study of hospitalized patients in Italy compared 334 inpatients with psoriasis to 338 inpatient controls with other skin disease. In subjects over 40 years of age, the metabolic syndrome was more prevalent among psoriatic patients than controls (OR = 1.65). Furthermore, psoriasis cases maintained higher individual rates of abdominal obesity and hypertriglyceridemia. Of interest, prevalence of hypertension, hyperglycemia, and abnormal high-density lipoprotein levels were similar in cases and controls. Notably, severity of psoriasis did not correlate with prevalence of metabolic syndrome[14].

A population-based study of patients from the UK presented similar findings[13]. With the same database used to show an association with MI (see above), investigators queried the records of over 127,000 patients with mild psoriasis (i.e. those never having received systemic therapy) and 3,800 with severe disease for risk factors for MI, including many components of the metabolic syndrome. Compared to matched controls, patients with mild psoriasis were more likely to be obese (OR = 1.27), hypertensive (OR = 1.03), hyperlipidemic (OR = 1.16), and diabetic (OR = 1.13). Patients with severe disease maintained an even greater propensity toward diabetes (OR = 1.62) and obesity (OR = 1.7), although results for hypertension and hyperlipidemia were not significant in this group.

Recently, researchers found higher levels of high-density lipoprotein (HDL), a well-known deterrent of atherosclerosis, among 200 patients at the time of diagnosis of psoriasis compared to age-matched controls[24]. Investigators speculate that this unexpected finding may illustrate compensation for elevations in very low-density lipoprotein (VLDL), an atherogenic molecule, also demonstrated among participants with psoriasis.

Under the direction of the International Psoriasis Council, a recent, interdisciplinary conference involving dermatologists, hepatologists, cardiologists, and others produced an intriguing dialog about the potential common pathophysiologic mechanisms of psoriasis and metabolic disease, such as obesity. Panelists reviewed epidemiologic and immunologic factors linking psoriasis to obesity. Connections to cardiovascular and liver disease were also discussed. A concise and thorough report from the conference with a listing of recommended prospective studies, was recently published by Sterry *et al.*[25].

GASTROINTESTINAL DISEASE
Steatohepatitis and hepatic fibrosis
General description
Marked by deposition of lipid globules and parenchymal inflammation, steatohepatitis describes a reaction of the liver to noxious insults or processes rather than a distinct disease[26]. The pathological state results from a variety of mechanisms: excessive alcohol consumption, drug toxicity, and metabolic derangement such as insulin resistance and obesity. Disproportionately affected by each of these, psoriasis sufferers seem ill-fated to develop this condition.

The pathologic cornerstone of steatohepatitis is macrovesicular steatosis, collections of intercellular lipid throughout the lobule signifying degeneration of parenchyma[26]. Other hallmarks of histology include a mixed inflammatory infiltrate and ballooning degeneration or necrosis of hepatocytes. Risk for progression to fibrosis and ultimately cirrhosis depends on the inciting insult(s). Among psoriasis patients treated with methotrexate, for example, 73% of patients developed hepatic fibrosis if daily alcohol consumption exceeds 15 g (i.e. about 19 ml) compared to 26% if intake is less, according to a broad meta-analysis[27].

Unfortunately, clinical and laboratory assessments inconsistently reflect histological progression of steatohepatitis, especially in psoriasis patients on methotrexate[28]. Liver biochemical tests and physical examination may be normal despite advanced hepatic fibrosis. Although typically absent, symptoms may include vague pain in the right upper quadrant, as well as fatigue. The liver may be enlarged and firm on abdominal palpation. Elevations in alanine aminotransferase (ALT) and aspartate aminotransferase (AST) rarely exceed 10-fold normal. Further, AST to ALT ratio reflects the insulting process, classically 2:1 for alcohol and less than one for nonalcoholic fatty liver disease (NAFLD)[24]. Methotrexate fails to demonstrate a consistent pattern of elevation of liver enzymes[29].

According to a recent study, ultrasound and computed tomography (CT) maintain high sensitivity (100%) and specificity (93%) for the detection of simple steatosis of the liver[30]. However, neither reliably distinguished steatosis from more advanced steatohepatitis.

Risk factors
Psoriasis sufferers experience a variety of insults to the liver, toxic and metabolic, that confer risk for the development of steatohepatitis. Paramount among them, alcohol consumption bestows risk of liver disease for men drinking 40–80 g (i.e. about 50–100 ml) daily over 12 years and for women consuming 20–40 g (i.e. about 25–50 ml) daily[31]. Indeed, alcoholic cirrhosis is relatively common among psoriatics[32]. Obesity, particularly intra-abdominal fat, correlates with degree of hepatic steatosis[33]. Other constituents of the metabolic syndrome, common among psoriatics as described above, impart risk of steatohepatitis as well. Type II diabetes increases the likelihood of the condition two-fold and resultant liver disease may follow an aggressive course[34]. Hyperlipidemia also correlates with steatohepatitis[26]. Indeed, psoriasis itself may independently predispose to the condition, particularly in the setting of methotrexate therapy (see below).

Methotrexate toxicity

A well-known hepatotoxin, methotrexate has been used to treat psoriasis since the 1950s[35]. A survey in 1974 revealed that 52% of dermatologists prescribed the folic acid antagonist for severe disease[36], a figure that increased to 58% in 1987[7]. Methotrexate causes hepatic fibrosis both via progressive steatosis and directly through damage to nonparenchymal stellate cells[29]. Unfortunately, methotrexate has been shown to induce greater hepatic injury to psoriasis sufferers than to those with RA, by 2.5- to 5-fold[27].

Several large studies have assessed the presence and progression of liver disease among psoriasis patients on methotrexate. In 1973, 81 patients with psoriasis underwent liver biopsy before and after treatment[37]. At cumulative doses greater than 2.2 g, hepatic fibrosis was more common but cirrhosis was not. Overall, cirrhosis developed in 3% of patients, a figure mirrored by later work in Texas and Canada[28,38]. Two studies from Scandinavia revealed a dose-dependent increase in occurrence of fibrosis and ultimately cirrhosis[39,40]. With large cumulative doses (> 4 g), cirrhosis developed in 10 and 21% of patients, respectively.

Indeed, some experts advocate liver biopsies only after cumulative doses > 4 g, in patients without risk factors for liver disease[41]. Furthermore, rheumatologists' guidelines for monitoring of methotrexate differ from dermatologists'. Specifically, data from the rheumatology literature suggest that, in the absence of other risk factors, liver biopsies are unnecessary if five of nine measures of serum transaminases are normal in a given year[42]. Fortunately, cirrhosis caused by methotrexate follows a relatively mild clinical course[39,43,44]. All in all, the risk of cirrhosis remains low with a cumulative dose of methotrexate less than 3–4 g, in the absence of other risk factors[45,46].

In response to the mounting evidence against liver biopsies in low-risk patients, the European Academy of Dermatology and Venereology and the American Academy of Dermatology recently released guidelines substantially altering the approach to liver biopsy in psoriasis patients on methotrexate[47, 48].

In patients without significant risk factors, guidelines for liver biopsy have been made much less stringent. In the absence of persistent laboratory abnormalities, liver biopsy should be deferred until a cumulative dose of 3.5–4 g of methotrexate is reached, a striking departure from the 1–1.5 g threshold endorsed previously.

Patients at risk for liver disease may be candidates for earlier biopsy. These include those with a history of moderate/excessive alcohol consumption, chronic hepatitis B or C, diabetes mellitus, obesity, hyperlipidemia, exposure to hepatotoxic drugs, and/or family members with heritable liver disease. For these patients, liver biopsy may be considered after 2–6 months of treatment course or at a cumulative methotrexate dose of 1–1.5 g, and every 1–1.5 g thereafter. A significant increase in transaminases may also prompt earlier liver biopsies if maintenance of methotrexate therapy is desired.

Surrogate markers for hepatic fibrosis may minimize, or potentially eliminate, the need for liver biopsy in the near future. The most promising marker, a serum assay for the amino-terminal peptide of procollagen III, demonstrates impressive sensitivity and has significantly reduced liver biopsies in psoriasis patients treated with methotrexate across several European centers[49]. The assay is widely available in Europe but is not yet commercially available in the USA. Novel radiographic techniques, such as a form of ultrasound known as transient elastography, may prove even more sensitive and specific for fibrosis, further reducing and possibly eliminating the role of liver biopsy in methotrexate-treated psoriasis patients[50].

Crohn's disease

As scientists further refine the genetic basis of psoriasis, overlap with other complex diseases emerges. Recently, geneticists discovered that a region on the long arm of chromosome 16 known to be associated with psoriasis, PSORS 8, also contains a susceptibility locus for Crohn's disease[51]. Additionally, Crohn's may share genetic linkage with psoriatic arthritis[52]. Although not well studied, an epidemiologic association appears to exist as well, as Crohn's sufferers may be up to five times more likely to develop psoriasis than the general population[53–55]. Researchers speculate that TNF-α provides a common pathogenic link to both diseases, a notion supported by the efficacy of anti-TNF-α therapy in psoriasis and Crohn's disease[56].

NEUROLOGICAL DISORDERS

Multiple sclerosis

The development and success of the biologic agents in the treatment of psoriasis raise inevitable concern about uncovering rare toxicities. Etanercept and infliximab appear to confer a small, albeit controversial, risk for demyelination resembling multiple sclerosis (MS)[57–60]. Among the 19 patients with psoriasis who have developed demyelination while on these drugs, symptoms tend to resolve with cessation of therapy. Evidence of successful resumption of biologics also exists[61]. There is evidence to suggest that a relationship between MS and psoriasis exists independently of treatment[62].

NEOPLASTIC DISEASE

Lymphoma

Several systemic treatments for psoriasis bestow risk for the development of lymphoma, including cyclosporin, methotrexate, and, to a much lesser extent, the biological agents[60,63,64]. Some argue that the disease itself, rather than the medications used to treat it, drives the increased risk (see below). Psoralen with UVA light, once thought to confer lymphoma risk, appears to do so only with concomitant methotrexate, according to a cohort study of 1,380 patients over 30 years[65]. Thus, whether psoriasis, a disease defined by immune system dysfunction, conveys risk independently of therapy still has to be addressed.

A recent population-based study from the UK followed a cohort of 3,994 patients with severe psoriasis, defined as those on systemic therapy, and 149,203 patients with mild disease for development of lymphoma[66]. Interestingly, both groups demonstrated increased relative risk (RR), greatest for Hodgkin's disease (RR = 3.18 and 1.42) and cutaneous T-cell lymphoma (RR = 10.75 and 4.1). The absolute risk attributable to psoriasis remains low, however, as these malignancies are generally uncommon.

PSYCHIATRIC DISORDERS

Depression

Chapter 8 documents the ravaging effects of psoriasis on quality of life. As expected, psoriatics experience symptoms of depression with alarming prevalence. In a recent study of 5,000 Italian patients with psoriasis, 62% of participants report depressive symptoms using a validated questionnaire[67]. Men less than 40 years of age without higher education demonstrate the highest rates. Sadly, thoughts of suicide also prevail among psoriasis sufferers and correlate with self-ratings of skin disease severity, according to a study of 217 patients in 1993[68]. Nearly 10% of these patients wished to be dead. Equally disturbing, healthcare professionals may not adequately assess for depressive symptoms among psoriasis patients, as recent work reveals that dermatologists fail to identify and discuss symptoms of anxiety and/or depression in 61% of distressed patients[69].

Excessive consumption of alcohol

In a population prone to depression, alcohol abuse often prevails. Indeed, research over the last 20 years demonstrates that excessive alcohol consumption is not only prevalent among psoriasis sufferers, but may also confer risk for the development of skin disease. A large cohort study from Sweden, for example, revealed that psoriasis associates with alcoholism and cirrhosis[70]. Prevalence of alcoholism in another large study of psoriatics was 11% compared to 3% in controls[71]. Compelling work published in the UK calculated an odds ratio of 8.01 for alcohol as an independent risk factor for the development of psoriasis[72]. When researchers stratify subjects according to gender, however, alcohol remains a risk factor for men[73], but not women[74]. Interestingly, both sexes report exacerbations of skin disease with heavy alcohol intake.

MORTALITY

Given the toll psoriasis exacts on the skin and other organ systems, it follows that overall mortality may be increased among those affected. In a recent, population-based cohort study of psoriatics in the UK, disturbing data revealed that patients with severe disease, defined by having received systemic therapy, maintained a higher mortality risk than matched controls[75]. This effect persisted even after controlling for inflammatory joint disease, known to increase mortality (see Chapter 4, Psoriatic arthritis). On average, lifespan was 3.5 years shorter for men and 4.4 years shorter for women with severe disease. Interestingly, mild disease, defined as no history of systemic therapy, had no effect on mortality.

CONCLUSION

Unfortunately, cross-sectional studies prohibit inferences of causality. In the many cases cited above, uncertainty persists as to whether a given disease predisposes to psoriasis or vice versa. Nevertheless, robust associations do exist. The list of concerns for psoriasis sufferers and for the healthcare personnel who care for them continues to grow.

It is incumbent on the psoriasis research community to initiate prospective studies, in addition to multiple drug- and country-specific registries, to discern the exact relationship of these comorbidities and risk factors with psoriasis. Whether diet and exercise modification in the generally overweight/obese population with moderate-to-severe psoriasis will reduce these factors must also be evaluated. The International Psoriasis Council is taking the lead on these and other issues, in consultation with specialists in the field of obesity, heart and liver disease, and diabetes, with major implications for the general well-being of the psoriasis population at large.

8 APPENDIX

ASSESSMENT TOOLS

PSORIASIS AREA AND SEVERITY INDEX (PASI)

Body area	Erythema (E) 0–4*	Induration (I) 0–4*	Scale (S) 0–4*	(I) Sum E + I + S	(II) Involvement 0–6**	(III) Product I × II	(IV) Multiplier	(V) Product III × IV
Head							0.1	
Upper limbs							0.2	
Trunk							0.3	
Lower limbs							0.4	
						Sum of column V = **PASI**		

* Erythema, induration, and scale: **0**, clear; **1**, slight; **2**, mild; **3**, moderate; **4**, severe

** Degree of psoriatic involvement: **0**, 0% (clear); **1**, <10%; **2**, 10–30%; **3**, 30%–50%; **4**, 50–70% ; **5**, 70–90% affected; **6**, 90–100%

1 **PASI.** To calculate the PASI, the sum of the severity rating for the three main signs (erythema, induration, and scale) is multiplied by the degree of involvement of the area affected. This product is then multiplied by a factor for each area and the results are added together to give the overall PASI score.

PHYSICIAN'S GLOBAL ASSESSMENT (PGA)

Severe	Severe – moderate	Moderate	Moderate – mild	Mild	Almost clear	Clear
1 ☐	2 ☐	3 ☐	4 ☐	5 ☐	6 ☐	7 ☐

Severe: very marked plaque elevation, scaling, and/or erythema
Severe to moderate: marked plaque elevation, scaling and/or erythema
Moderate: moderate plaque elevation, scaling, and/or erythema
Moderate to mild: intermediate between evaluation scores 3 and 5
Mild: slight plaque elevation scaling, and/or erythema
Almost clear: intermediate between evaluation scores 5 and 7
Clear: no signs of psoriasis (post-inflammatory hypopigmentation or hyperpigmentation may be present)

2 **PGA.** The healthcare provider judges severity of the affected patient's disease using a scale from 1–7, with a lower score indicating greater severity.

PSORIASIS DISABILITY INDEX (PDI)

Thank you for your help in completing this questionnaire.

Please tick one box for every question. Every question relates to the *last four weeks only*.

Daily activities		Very much	A lot	A little	Not at all
1	How much has your psoriasis interfered with you carrying out work around the house or garden?	❑	❑	❑	❑
2	How often have you worn different types or colours of clothes because of your psoriasis?	❑	❑	❑	❑
3	How much more have you had to change or wash your clothes?	❑	❑	❑	❑
4	How much of a problem has your psoriasis been at the hairdressers?	❑	❑	❑	❑
5	How much has your psoriasis resulted in you having to take more baths than usual?	❑	❑	❑	❑

There are two different versions of questions 6, 7 and 8. If you are at regular work or at school please answer the first set of questions. If you are not at work or school please answer the second set of questions.

Work or school		Very much	A lot	A little	Not at all
6	How much has your psoriasis made you lose time off work or school over the last four weeks?	❑	❑	❑	❑
7	How much has your psoriasis prevented you from doing things at work or school over the last four weeks?	❑	❑	❑	❑
8	Has your career been affected by your psoriasis, e.g. promotion refused, lost a job, asked to change a job?	❑	❑	❑	❑

If not at work or school		Very much	A lot	A little	Not at all
6	How much has your psoriasis stopped you carrying out your normal daily activities over the last four weeks?	❑	❑	❑	❑
7	How much has your psoriasis altered the way in which you carry out your normal daily activities over the last four weeks?	❑	❑	❑	❑
8	Has your career been affected by your psoriasis, e.g. promotion refused, lost a job, asked to change a job?	❑	❑	❑	❑

Personal relationships		Very much	A lot	A little	Not at all
9	Has your psoriasis resulted in sexual difficulties over the last four weeks?	❑	❑	❑	❑
10	Has your psoriasis created problems with your partner or any of your close friends or relatives?	❑	❑	❑	❑

3 PDI. The PDI is calculated by summing the score of each of the 15 questions on a scale of 0–3. The higher the score, the more quality of life is impaired. The PDI can also be expressed as a percentage of the maximum possible score of 45.

© A Y Finlay 1993

PDI cont.

Leisure	Very much	A lot	A little	Not at all
11 How much has your psoriasis stopped you going out socially or to any special functions?	❑	❑	❑	❑
12 Is your psoriasis making it difficult for you to do any sport?	❑	❑	❑	❑
13 Have you been unable to use, criticized for or stopped from using communal bathing or changing facilities?	❑	❑	❑	❑
14 Has your psoriasis resulted in you smoking or drinking alcohol more than you would do normally?	❑	❑	❑	❑

Treatment	Very much	A lot	A little	Not at all
15 To what extent has your psoriasis or treatment made your home messy or untidy?	❑	❑	❑	❑

ACR RESPONSE CRITERIA FOR RHEUMATOID ARTHRITIS CLINICAL TRIALS (ACR-20)

20% improvement in:

1	Swollen joints	+/–
2	Tender joints	+/–

And 3 of following 5:

3	Physician's global assessment	+/–
4	Patient's global assessment	+/–
5	Functional status or physical disability	+/–
6	Acute phase reactants (ESR or CRP)*	+/–
7	Radiographs	+/–

* CRP, C-reactive protein; ESR, erythrocyte sedimentation rate.

4 ACR-20. The American College of Rheumatology criteria assess efficacy of treatment. For the purposes of clinical trials in RA, a 'responder' to treatment exhibits 20% improvement in (1) and (2), as well as three of the remaining five (3–7).

5 PsAQoL. A patient-reported, 20-item assessment tool specfic to psoriatic arthritis.

PSORIATIC ARTHRITIS-SPECIFIC QUALITY OF LIFE INSTRUMENT (PsAQoL)

1	I feel tired whatever I do	❑
2	I find it difficult to have a good wash	❑
3	It's too much effort to go out and see people	❑
4	I feel there's no enjoyment in my life	❑
5	I feel I am losing my independence	❑
6	I often get angry with myself	❑
7	I can't do the things I want to do	❑
8	I feel older than my years	❑
9	I'm unable to join in activities with my friends or family	❑
10	It limits the places I can go	❑
11	I have to push myself to do things	❑
12	I am easily irritated by other people	❑
13	I have to keep stopping what I'm doing to rest	❑
14	I feel dependent on others	❑
15	It takes me a long time to get going in the morning	❑
16	I take it out on people close to me	❑
17	I can't do things on the spur of the moment	❑
18	I feel like a prisoner in my own home	❑
19	I have to limit what I do each day	❑
20	It puts a strain on my personal relationships	❑

KOO–MENTER PSORIASIS INSTRUMENT (KMPI)

| PATIENT SELF-ASSESSMENT | Name: | | | | | | | | | Date: | | |

Part 1: Quality of life

Please answer each of the following questions as they pertain to your psoriasis *during the past month*.
(Circle one number per question.)

1	How **self-conscious** do you feel with regard to your psoriasis?	0	1	2	3	4	5	6	7	8	9	10
2	How **helpless** do you feel with regard to your psoriasis?	0	1	2	3	4	5	6	7	8	9	10
3	How **embarrassed** do you feel with regard to your psoriasis?	0	1	2	3	4	5	6	7	8	9	10
4	How **angry** or **frustrated** do you feel with regard to your psoriasis?	0	1	2	3	4	5	6	7	8	9	10
5	To what extent does your psoriasis make your **appearance** unsightly?	0	1	2	3	4	5	6	7	8	9	10
6	How **disfiguring** is your psoriasis?	0	1	2	3	4	5	6	7	8	9	10
7	How much does your psoriasis impact on your overall **emotional well-being**?	0	1	2	3	4	5	6	7	8	9	10
8	To what extent does your psoriasis interfere with your capacity to **enjoy life**?	0	1	2	3	4	5	6	7	8	9	10

How much have each of the following been affected by your psoriasis *during the past month*.
(Circle one number per question.)

9	Itching?	0	1	2	3	4	5	6	7	8	9	10
10	Physical irritation?	0	1	2	3	4	5	6	7	8	9	10
11	Physical pain or soreness?	0	1	2	3	4	5	6	7	8	9	10
12	Choice of clothing to conceal psoriasis?	0	1	2	3	4	5	6	7	8	9	10

Part 2

Using the figures below, place an 'X' on the parts of your body that *currently* have psoriasis.

Part 3

A. Have you ever been diagnosed with psoriatic arthritis?   Yes ❑   No ❑

B. Do you have swollen, tender, or stiff joints (e.g. hands, feet, hips, back)?   Yes ❑   No ❑

If yes, how many joints are affected?

1 ❑   2 ❑   3 ❑   4 ❑   More ❑

If yes, how much have your joint symptoms affected your day-to-day activities?

Not at all ❑   A little ❑   A lot ❑   Very much ❑

☆ *Once completed, please return to medical staff.*

6 KMPI. Questionnaires for both patient and physician to assess the impact of psoriasis on quality of life and determine which patients are most likely to benefit from systemic therapy.

KMPI cont.

PHYSICIAN ASSESSMENT   Name: Date:

Part 1: Total Quality-of-Life assessment score (from Part 1 of previous page)

Part 2: Area of involvement – % BSA (body surface area)

Head	[ ] %	up to 9% of total BSA
Anterior trunk	[ ] %	up to 18% of total BSA
Posterior trunk	[ ] %	up to 18% of total BSA
Right leg	[ ] %	up to 18% of total BSA (includes buttock)
Left leg	[ ] %	up to 18% of total BSA (includes buttock)
Both arms	[ ] %	up to 18% of total BSA
Genitalia	[ ] %	1% of total BSA
Total BSA	[ ] %	

Note: Patient's open hand (from wrist to tip of fingers) with fingers together and thumb tucked to the side equals approximately 1% of body surface area.

Part 3: In terms of psoriasis severity, does the patient have:

Plaque, erythrodermic, or pustular psoriasis with >10% BSA involvement?	Yes ☐	No ☐
Guttate psoriasis?	Yes ☐	No ☐
Localized (<10% BSA) psoriasis but resistant to optimized attempts at topical therapy or physically disabling (e.g. palmarplantar psoriasis)?	Yes ☐	No ☐
Localized (<10% BSA) but serious subtype with possibility of progression (e.g. pustular or pre-erythrodermic psoriasis)?	Yes ☐	No ☐
Clinical evidence of psoriatic joint disease as assessed by physician (e.g. examine IP, MCP, and MT joints of hands, wrists, feet, and ankles, plus patient responses from Part 3 of patient self-assessment)?	Yes ☐	No ☐
Substantial psychosocial or quality-of-life impact documented by patient Quality-of-Life self-assessment score of ≥50?	Yes ☐	No ☐

Part 4: Is phototherapy an option?

Is a suitable phototherapy unit readily accessible to the patient?	Yes ☐	No ☐
Does the anatomical location or form of psoriasis (e.g. scalp, inverse, erythrodermic) preclude phototherapy?	Yes ☐	No ☐
Does the patient have the dedication, time, stamina, or transportation for phototherapy?	Yes ☐	No ☐
Has phototherapy, as monotherapy, failed in the past?	Yes ☐	No ☐
Is phototherapy contraindicated (e.g. photosensitive drugs, history of multiple skin cancers)?	Yes ☐	No ☐
In your clinical judgment, is phototherapy likely to yield substantial improvement to justify its use before systemic therapy?	Yes ☐	No ☐

Physician/nurse comments:

If at least one of the shaded boxes in both Part 3 and Part 4 above are checked, then the patient is a candidate for systemic therapy.

CONCLUSION: The patient is a candidate for systemic therapy   Yes ☐   No ☐

SF-36 HEALTH SURVEY

INSTRUCTIONS: This set of questions asks for your views about your health. This information will help keep track of how you feel and how well you are able to do your usual activities. Answer every question by marking the answer as indicated. If you are unsure about how to answer a question please give the best answer you can.

1	In general, would you say your health is: (Please tick **one** box.)		
		Excellent	❏
		Very good	❏
		Good	❏
		Fair	❏
		Poor	❏

2	*Compared to one year ago*, how would you rate your health in general *now*? (Please tick **one** box.)		
		Much better than one year ago	❏
		Somewhat better now than one year ago	❏
		About the same as one year ago	❏
		Somewhat worse now than one year ago	❏
		Much worse now than one year ago	❏

3 The following questions are about activities you might do during a typical day. Does *your health now limit you* in these activities? If so, how much? (**Please circle one number on each line.**)

	Activities	Limited a lot	Limited a little	Not limited at all
3a	**Vigorous activities** such as running, lifting heavy objects, participating in strenuous sports	1	2	3
3b	**Moderate activities**, such as moving a table, pushing a vacuum cleaner, bowling, or playing golf	1	2	3
3c	Lifting or carrying groceries	1	2	3
3d	Climbing **several** flights of stairs	1	2	3
3e	Climbing **one** flight of stairs	1	2	3
3f	Bending, kneeling, or stooping	1	2	3
3g	Walking **more than a mile**	1	2	3
3h	Walking **several blocks**	1	2	3
3i	Walking **one block**	1	2	3
3j	Bathing or dressing yourself	1	2	3

4 During the *past 4 weeks*, have you had any of the following problems with your work or other regular daily activities *as a result of your physical health*?

	(**Please circle one number on each line.**)	Yes	No
4a	Cut down on the **amount of time** you spent on work or other activities	1	2
4b	Accomplished **less** than you would like	1	2
4c	Were **limited** in the **kind** of work or other activities	1	2
4d	Had **difficulty** performing the work or other activities (for example, it took extra effort)	1	2

5 During the *past 4 weeks*, have you had any of the following problems with your work or other regular daily activities *as a result of any emotional problems* (e.g. feeling depressed or anxious)?

	(**Please circle one number on each line.**)	Yes	No
5a	Cut down on the **amount of time** you spent on work or other activities	1	2
5b	Accomplished **less** than you would like	1	2
5c	Didn't do work or other activities as **carefully** as usual	1	2

SF-36 cont:

6	During the *past 4 weeks*, to what extent has your physical health or emotional problems interfered with your normal social activities with family, friends, neighbors, or groups? (Please tick **one** box.)	Not at all	☐
		Slightly	☐
		Moderately	☐
		Quite a bit	☐
		Extremely	☐
7	How much *physical* pain have you had during the *past 4 weeks*? (Please tick **one** box.)	None	☐
		Very mild	☐
		Mild	☐
		Moderate	☐
		Severe	☐
		Very severe	☐
8	During the *past 4 weeks*, how much did *pain* interfere with your normal work (including both work outside the home and housework)? (Please tick **one** box.)	Not at all	☐
		A bit	☐
		Moderately	☐
		Quite a bit	☐
		Extremely	☐

9 These questions are about how you feel and how things have been with you during the *past 4 weeks*. Please give the one answer that is closest to the way you have been feeling for each item.

(Please circle one number on each line.)	All of the time	Most of the time	A lot of the time	Some of the time	A little of the time	None of the time
9a Did you feel full of life?	1	2	3	4	5	6
9b Have you been a very nervous person?	1	2	3	4	5	6
9c Have you felt so down in the dumps that nothing could cheer you up?	1	2	3	4	5	6
9d Have you felt calm and peaceful?	1	2	3	4	5	6
9e Did you have a lot of energy?	1	2	3	4	5	6
9f Have you felt downhearted and blue?	1	2	3	4	5	6
9g Did you feel worn out?	1	2	3	4	5	6
9h Have you been a happy person?	1	2	3	4	5	6
9i Did you feel tired?	1	2	3	4	5	6

10	During the *past 4 weeks*, how much of the time has your *physical health or emotional problems* interfered with your social activities (like visiting with friends, relatives etc.) (Please tick **one** box.)	All of the time	☐
		Most of the time	☐
		Some of the time	☐
		A little of the time	☐
		None of the time	☐

11 How **true** or **false** is *each* of the following statements for you?

(Please circle one number on each line.)	Definitely true	Mostly true	Don't know	Mostly false	Definitely false
11a I seem to get sick a little easier than other people	1	2	3	4	5
11b I am as healthy as anybody I know	1	2	3	4	5
11c I expect my health to get worse	1	2	3	4	5
11d My health is excellent	1	2	3	4	5

7   SF-36®. This is a generic, short-form survey, with 36 questions covering eight measures of health: physical functioning, role–physical, bodily pain, general health, vitality, social functioning, role–emotional, and mental health.

© *Medical Outcomes Trust*

STANFORD HEALTH ASSESSMENT QUESTIONNAIRE (HAQ)

DISABILITY INDEX AND PAIN SCALE

In this section we are interested in learning how your illness affects your ability to function in daily life. Please check the response which best describes your usual abilities *over the past week*

Dressing and grooming	Without **any** difficulty	With **some** difficulty	With **much** difficulty	**Unable** to do
Are you able to:				
Dress yourself, including tying shoelaces and doing buttons?	❑	❑	❑	❑
Shampoo your hair?	❑	❑	❑	❑
Arising				
Are you able to:				
Stand up from a straight chair?	❑	❑	❑	❑
Get in and out of bed?	❑	❑	❑	❑
Eating				
Are you able to:				
Cut your meat?	❑	❑	❑	❑
Lift a full glass or cup to your mouth?	❑	❑	❑	❑
Open a new milk carton?	❑	❑	❑	❑
Walking				
Are you able to:				
Walk outdoors on flat ground?	❑	❑	❑	❑
Climb up five steps?	❑	❑	❑	❑

Please check any **aids** or **devices** that you usually use for any of these activities:

❑ Cane
❑ Walker
❑ Crutches
❑ Wheelchair

❑ Devices used for dressing (button hook, zipper pull, long-handled shoe horn, etc.)
❑ Built-up or special utensils
❑ Special or built-up chair
❑ Other (specify:_____)

Please check any categories for which you usually need **help from another person**:

❑ Dressing and grooming
❑ Arising

❑ Eating
❑ Walking

8 HAQ disability index and pain scale. This shows the first two domains of the full HAQ, which also measures drug side-effects and monetary costs. Disability is assessed by the eight categories of dressing, arising, eating, walking, hygiene, reach, grip, and common activities; discomfort is determined by the presence of pain and its severity.

© *Stanford University School of Medicine, Division of Immunology & Rheumatology*

HAQ cont.

Please check the response which best describes your usual abilities *over the past week*.

Hygiene	Without **any** difficulty	With **some** difficulty	With **much** difficulty	**Unable** to do
Are you able to:				
Wash and dress your body?	❑	❑	❑	❑
Take a tub bath?	❑	❑	❑	❑
Get on and off the toilet?	❑	❑	❑	❑
Reach				
Are you able to:				
Reach and get down a 5-lb object (e.g. a bag of sugar) from just above your head?	❑	❑	❑	❑
Bend down to pick up clothing from the floor?	❑	❑	❑	❑
Grip				
Are you able to:				
Open car doors?	❑	❑	❑	❑
Open jars which have been previously opened?	❑	❑	❑	❑
Turn faucets on and off?	❑	❑	❑	❑
Activities				
Are you able to:				
Run errands and shop?	❑	❑	❑	❑
Get in and out of a car?	❑	❑	❑	❑
Do chores such as vacuuming or yardwork?	❑	❑	❑	❑

Please check any **aids** or **devices** that you usually use for any of these activities:

❑ Raised toilet seat   ❑ Bathtub bar
❑ Bathtub seat   ❑ Long-handled appliances for reach
❑ Jar opener (for jars previously opened)   ❑ Long-handled appliances for bathroom
❑ Other (specify:_____)

Please check any categories for which you usually need **help from another person**:

❑ Hygiene   ❑ Gripping and opening things
❑ Reach   ❑ Errands and chores

We are also intrested in learning whether or not you are affected by pain because of your illness.
How much pain have you had because of your illness *in the past week*?
Place a vertical mark (I) on the line to indicate the severity of the pain.

No pain   Severe pain

0   100

Considering all the ways your illness affects you, rate how you are doing on the following scale
by placing a vertical mark (I) on the line.

Very well   Very poor

0   100

DERMATOLOGY LIFE QUALITY INDEX (DLQI)

Hospital No:	Date:	Score:
Name:	Diagnosis:	
Address:		

The aim of this questionnaire is to measure how much your skin problem has affected your life *over the last week*. Please tick one box for each question.

1   Over the last week, how **itchy, sore, painful** or **stinging** has your skin been?

- Very much ❑
- A lot ❑
- A little ❑
- Not at all ❑

2   Over the last week, how **embarrassed** or **self-conscious** have you been because of your skin?

- Very much ❑
- A lot ❑
- A little ❑
- Not at all ❑

3   Over the last week, how much has your skin interfered with you going **shopping** or looking after your **home** or **garden**?

- Very much ❑
- A lot ❑
- A little ❑
- Not at all ❑   Not relevant ❑

4   Over the last week, how much has your skin influenced the **clothes** you wear?

- Very much ❑
- A lot ❑
- A little ❑
- Not at all ❑   Not relevant ❑

5   Over the last week, how much has your skin affected any **social** or **leisure** activities?

- Very much ❑
- A lot ❑
- A little ❑
- Not at all ❑   Not relevant ❑

6   Over the last week, how much has your skin made it difficult for you to do any **sport**?

- Very much ❑
- A lot ❑
- A little ❑
- Not at all ❑   Not relevant ❑

7   Over the last week, has your skin prevented you from **working** or **studying**?

- Yes ❑
- No ❑   Not relevant ❑

If 'No', over the last week how much has your skin been a problem at **work** or **studying**?

- A lot ❑
- A little ❑
- Not at all ❑

8   Over the last week, how much has your skin created problems with your **partner** or any of your **close friends** or **relatives**?

- Very much ❑
- A lot ❑
- A little ❑
- Not at all ❑   Not relevant ❑

9   Over the last week, how much has your skin caused any **sexual difficulties**?

- Very much ❑
- A lot ❑
- A little ❑
- Not at all ❑   Not relevant ❑

10   Over the last week, how much of a problem has the **treatment** for your skin been, for example by making your home messy, or by taking up time?

- Very much ❑
- A lot ❑
- A little ❑
- Not at all ❑   Not relevant ❑

9   **DLQI**. The first dermatology-specific QOL instrument. © *AY Finlay, GK Khan, April 1992*.

ABBREVIATIONS

ACR	American College of Rheumatology
ACR-20	American College of Rheumatology – 20% responder criteria
AD	atopic dermatitis
ALT	alanine aminotransferase
APC	antigen-presenting cell
AST	aspartate aminotransferase
BB	broadband
BSA	body surface area
CCHCR-1	coiled-coil α-helical rod protein 1
CD	cluster of differentiation
CLA	cutaneous lymphocyte antigen
CT	computed tomography
CTCL	cutaneous T-cell lymphoma
DC	dendritic cell
DIP	distal–interphalangeal (joint)
DLQI	Dermatology Life Quality Index
DM	diabetes mellitus
ESR	erythrocyte sedimentation rate
FDA	Food and Drug Administration
HAQ	Health Assessment Questionnaire
HDL	high-density lipoprotein
HLA	human leukocyte antigen
HPV	human papilloma virus
HRQOL	health-related quality of life
HTN	hypertension
ICAM-1	intercellular adhesion molecule-1
ICAMs	intercellular adhesion molecules
IFN-α	interferon alpha
IFN-γ	interferon gamma
IL-2	interleukin 2
iNOS	inducible nitric oxide synthase
KIR	killer-cell immunoglobulin-like receptor
KMPI	Koo–Menter Psoriasis Instrument
KOH	potassium hydroxide
LAMP	lysosomal-associated membrane protein
MCP	metacarpal–phalangeal (joint)
MED	minimum erythema dosage
MHC	major histocompatibility complex
MI	myocardial infarction
MLR	mixed lymphocyte response
MRI	magnetic resonance imaging
MS	multiple sclerosis
MTX	methotrexate

NAFLD	nonalcoholic fatty liver disease
NB	narrowband
NKT	natural killer T cells
NSAID	nonsteroidal anti-inflammatory drug
OA	osteoarthritis
OMERACT	Outcome Measures in Rheumatoid Arthritis Clinical Trials
OR	odds ratio
PAS	periodic-acid Schiff
PASI	Psoriasis Area and Severity Index
pDC	plasmacytoid dendritic cells
PDI	Psoriasis Disability Index
PGA	Physician Global Assessment
PR	pityriasis rosea
PRP	pityriasis rubra pilaris
PsA	psoriatic arthritis
PsAQoL	Psoriatic Arthritis-specific Quality of Life instrument
PUVA	psoralen with ultraviolet A
RA	rheumatoid arthritis
RAPTOR	regulatory associated protein of mammalian target of rapamycin
RF	rheumatoid factor
RR	relative risk
SCCIS	squamous cell carcinoma *in situ*
SF-36	Short Form 36
SNP	single nucleotide polymorphism
SPI	Salford Psoriasis Index
STAT1	signal transducer and activator of transcription 1
TB	tuberculosis
TCR	T cell receptor
TLR	toll-like receptor
TNF-α	tumor necrosis factor alpha
VCAM-1	vascular adhesion molecule-1
VEGF	vascular endothelial growth factor
VLDL	very low-density lipoprotein

REFERENCES

Chapter 1

[1] Bechet PE (1936). Psoriasis, a brief historical review. *Archives of Dermatology and Syphilis* **33**: 327–334.

[2] Menter MA (2003). *Psoriasis: From Leprosy to Biologic Drug Development*. Waco, TX, Baylor University Medical Center Internal Medicine Grand Rounds.

[3] Celsus AC (1837). *De re medica*, 3rd edn (trans James Grieve). London, E. Portwine.

[4] Glickman FS (1986). Lepra, psora, psoriasis. *Journal of the American Academy of Dermatology* **14**:863–866.

[5] Willan R (1808). *On cutaneous diseases*. London, Johnson.

[6] Hebra F (1868). *On Disease of the Skin*, vol. II. London, New Syndenham Society.

[7] Milton JL (1972). *Diseases of the Skin*. London, Robert Hardwicke.

[8] Pusey WA (1933). *History of Dermatology*. Springfield, IL, Charles C. Thomas.

[9] Koebner H (1876). Zur Aetiologie der Psoriasis. *Viertel Jahresschrift fur Dermatologie und Syphilis* **8**:559–561.

[10] Munro WJ (1898). Note sur l'histopathologie du psoriasis. *Annales de Dermatologie et de Syphiligraphie* **9**: 961–967.

[11] von Zumbusch L (1910). Psoriasis und pustulöses exanthem. *Archives of Dermatology and Syphilis* **99**: 335.

[12] Woronoff DL (1926). Die peripheren Veranderungen der Haut um die Effloreszenzen der Psoriasis Vulgaris und *Syphilis Corymbosa*. *Dermatologische Wochenschrift* **82**: 249–258.

[13] Griffiths CE, Christophers E, Barker JN, *et al.* (2007). A classification of psoriasis vulgaris according to phenotype. *British Journal of Dermatology* **156**:258–262.

[14] National Psoriasis Foundation. Available from: www.psoriasis.org/about/stats/#3.

[15] Bell LM, Sedlack R, Beard MC, *et al.* (1991). Incidence of psoriasis in Rochester, Minn, 1980–1983. *Archives of Dermatology* **127**: 1184–1187.

[16] Gelfand JM (2005). Prevalence and treatment of psoriasis in the United Kingdom: A population-based study. *Archives of Dermatology* **141**: 1537–1541.

[17] Kidd CB, Meenan JC (1961). A dermatological survey of long-stay mental patients. *British Journal of Dermatology* **73**: 129–133.

[18] Rea JN, Newhouse ML, Halil T (1976). Skin disease in Lambeth. *British Journal of Preventive and Social Medicine* **30**: 107–114.

[19] Centers for Disease Control and Prevention, National Center for Health Statistics (2003). Vital and health statistics: Current estimates from the National Health Interview Survey, 1996. Atlanta, GA, Centers for Disease Control and Prevention, National Center for Health Statistics.

[20] Koo J (1995). Population-based epidemiology of psoriasis with emphasis on quality of life assessment. *Dermatologic Clinics* **14**: 485–496.

[21] Gelfand JM, Stern RS, Nijsten T, *et al.* (2005). The prevalence of psoriasis in African-Americans: Results from a population-based study. *Journal of the American Academy of Dermatology* **52**: 23–26.

[22] Obasi OE (1986). Psoriasis vulgaris in the Guinea Savanah region of Nigeria. *International Journal of Dermatology* **25**: 181–183.

[23] Convit J (1962). Investigation of the incidence of psoriasis among Latin American Indians. In: *Proceedings of the XIIth Congress on Dermatology*. Amsterdam, Exerpta Medica Foundation, p. 196.

[24] Farber EM, Nall ML (1998). Epidemiology: Natural history and genetics. In: *Psoriasis*. HH Roenigk, HI Maibach (eds). New York, Marcel Dekker, pp. 107–158.

[25] Yui Yip S (1984). The prevalence of psoriasis in the mongoloid race. *Journal of the American Academy of Dermatology* **10**: 965–968.

[26] Camp RDR (1998). Psoriasis. In: *Textbook of Dermatology*, 6th edn. RH Champion, JL Burton, DA Burns (eds). London, Blackwell Sciences, pp. 1589–1590.

[27] Holgate MC (1975). The age-of-onset of psoriasis. *British Journal of Dermatology* **92**: 443–448.

[28] Hellgren L (1967). *Psoriasis. The prevalence in sex, age, and occupational groups in total populations in Sweden. Morphology, inheritance, and association with other skin and rheumatic diseases*. Stockholm, Almqvist & Wiksell, pp. 19–53.

[29] Smith ES (2001). Demographics of aging and skin disease. *Clinics in Geriatric Medicine* **17**: 631–641.

[30] Henseler T, Christophers E (1985). Psoriasis of early and late onset: Characterization of two types of psoriasis vulgaris. *Journal of the American Academy of Dermatology* **13**: 450–456.

[31] Braathen LR, Botten G, Bjerkdal T (1989). Prevalence of psoriasis in Norway. *Acta Dermato-venereologica* **142** (Suppl.): 5–8.

[32] Duffy DL, Spelman LS, Martin NG (1993). Psoriasis in Australian twins. *Journal of the American Academy of Dermatology* **29**: 428–434.

[33] Snellman E, Lauharanta J, Reunanen A, *et al.* (1993). Effect of heliotherapy on skin and joint symptoms in psoriasis. A six-month follow-up study. *British Journal of Dermatology* **128**: 172–177.

[34] van de Kerkhof PCM (2003). Psoriasis. In: *Dermatology*. JL Bolognia, JL Jorizzo, RP Rapini (eds). Mosby, St Louis, pp. 125–149.

[35] Griffiths CEM, Barker JN (2007). Pathogenesis and clinical features of psoriasis. *Lancet* **370**:263–271.

[36] Liu Y, Helms C, Liao W, *et al.* (2008). A genome-wide association study of psoriasis and psoriatic arthritis identifies new disease loci. *PLoS Genetics* **4**: 1–14.

[37] Detmar M, Brown LF, Claffey KP, *et al.* (1994). Overexpression of vascular permeability factor/vascular endothelial growth factor and its receptors in psoriasis. *Journal of Experimental Medicine* **180**:1141–1146.

[38] Creamer D, Allen MH, Groves RW, Barker JNWN (1996). Circulating vascular permeability factor/vascular endothelial growth factor erythroderma. *Lancet* **348**: 1101.

[39] Xia YP, Li B, Hylton D, *et al.* (2003). Transgenic delivery of VEGF to mouse skin leads to an inflammatory condition resembling human psoriasis. *Blood* **102**: 161–168.

[40] Robert C, Kupper T (1999). Inflammatory skin diseases, T cells and immune surveillance. *New England Journal of Medicine* **341**:1817–1828.

[41] Prinz JC, Vollmer S, Boehncke WH, *et al.* (1999). Selection of conserved TCR VDJ rearrangements in chronic psoriatic plaques indicates a common antigen in psoriasis vulgaris. *European Journal of Immunology* **29**:3360–3368.

[42] Bonish B, Jullien D, Dutronc Y, *et al.* (2000). Overexpression of CD1d by keratinocytes in psoriasis and CD1d-dependent IFN-gamma production by NK-T cell. *Journal of Immunology* **165**: 4076–4085.

[43] Valdimarsson H, Baker BS, Jonsdottir I, *et al.* (1995). Psoriasis: A T-cell-mediated autoimmune disease induced by streptococcal superantigens? *Immunology Today* **16**: 145–149.

[44] Andressen C, Henseler T (1982). [Inheritance of psoriasis. Analysis of 2035 family histories.] *Hautarzt* **33**: 214–217.

[45] Farber EM, Nall NL, Watson W (1974). Natural history of psoriasis in 61 twin pairs. *Archives of Dermatology* **109**: 207–211.

[46] Bowcock AM, Krueger JG (2005). Getting under the skin: The immunogenetics of psoriasis. *Nature Reviews Immunology* **5**: 699–711.

[47] Capon F, Trembath RC, Barker JNWN (2004). An update on the genetics of psoriasis. *Dermatologic Clinics* **22**: 339–347.

[48] Trembath RC, Clough RL, Rosbotham JL, *et al.* (1997). Identification of a major susceptibility gene locus on chromosome 6p and evidence for further disease loci revealed by a two stage genome-wide search in psoriasis. *Human Molecular Genetics* **6**: 813–820.

[49] Curry JL, Qin JZ, Bonish B, *et al.* (2003). Innate immune-related receptors in normal and psoriatic skin. *Archives of Pathology and Laboratory Medicine* **127**: 178–186.

[50] Allen MH, Ameen M, Veal C, *et al.* (2005). The major psoriasis susceptibility locus PSORS1 is not a risk factor for late-onset psoriasis. *Journal of Investigative Dermatology* **124**: 103–107.

[51] Tiikikainen A, Lassus A, Karvonen J, *et al.* (1980). Psoriasis and HLA-Cw6. *British Journal of Dermatology* **102**: 179–184.

[52] Bowcock AM, Cookson WO (2004). The genetics of psoriasis, psoriatic arthritis and atopic dermatitis. *Human Molecular Genetics* **13**: R43–R55.

[53] Allen M, Ishida-Yamamoto A, McGrath JA, *et al.* (2001). Corneodesmosin expression in psoriasis vulgaris differs from normal skin and other inflammatory skin disorders. *Laboratory Investigation* **81**: 969–976.

[54] Tomfohrde J, Silverman J, Barnes R, *et al.* (1994). Gene for familial psoriasis susceptibility mapped to the distal end of human chromosome 17q. *Science* **264**: 1141–1145.

[55] Helms C, Cao L, Krueger JL, *et al.* (2003). A putative RUNX1 binding site variant between *SLC9A3R1* and *NAT9* is associated with susceptibility to psoriasis. *Nature Genetics* **35**: 349–356.

[56] Capon F, Helms C, Veal D, *et al.* (2004). Genetic analysis of PSORS2 markers in a UK dataset supports the association between RAPTOR SNP's and familial psoriasis. *Journal of Medical Genetics* **41**: 459–460.

[57] Broomley SK, Burack WR, Johnson KG, *et al.* (2001). The immunological synapse. *Annual Review of Immunology* **19**: 375–396.

[58] Davis SJ, Ikemizu S, Evans EJ, *et al.* (2003). The nature of molecular recognition by T cells. *Nature Immunology* **4**: 217–224.

[59] Capon F, Novelli G, Semprini S, *et al.* (1999). Searching for psoriasis susceptibility genes in Italy: genome scan and evidence for a new locus on chromosome 1. *Journal of Investigative Dermatology* **112**: 32–35.

[60] Bhalerao J, Bowcock AM (1998). The genetics of psoriasis: a complex disorder of the skin and immune system. *Human Molecular Genetics* **7**: 1537–1545.

[61] De Heller-Milev M, Huber M, Panizzon R, Hohl D (2000). Expression of small proline-rich proteins in neoplastic and inflammatory skin diseases. *British Journal of Dermatology* **143**: 733–740.

[62] Marshall D, Hardman MJ, Nield KM, Byrne C (2001). Differentially expressed late constituents of the epidermal cornified envelope. *Proceedings of the National Academy of Sciences of the United States of America* **98**: 13031–13036.

[63] Hewett D, Samuelsson L, Polding J, *et al.* (2002). Identification of a psoriasis susceptibility candidate gene by linkage disequilibrium mapping with a localized single nucleotide polymorphism map. *Genomics* **79**: 305–314.

[64] Hebert SC, Mount DB, Gamba G (2004). Molecular physiology of cation-coupled Cl-cotransport: SLC12 family. *Pflügers Archiv* **447**: 580–593.

[65] Mueller W, Hermann B (1979). Ciclosporin for psoriasis. *New England Journal of Medicine* **301**: 555.

[66] Ferenzi K, Burack L, Pope M, *et al.* (2000). CD69, HLA-DR, and IL-2R identify persistently activated T cells in psoriasis vulgaris lesional skin: Blood and skin comparisons by flow cytommetry. *Journal of Autoimmunity* **14**: 63–78.

[67] Sugiyama H, Gyulai R, Toichi E, *et al.* (2005). Dysfunctional blood and target tissue CD4+CD25high regulatory T cells in psoriasis: Mechanism underlying unrestrained pathogenic effector T cell proliferation. *Journal of Immunology* **174**: 164–173.

[68] Rottman JB, Smith TL, Ganley KG, *et al.* (2001). Potential role of chemokine receptors CXCR3, CCR4 and integrin a_Eb_7 in the pathogenesis of psoriasis vulgaris. *Laboratory Investigation* **81**: 335–347.

[69] Nickoloff BJ, Wrone-Smith T, Bonish B, Porcelli SA (1999). Response of murine and normal human skin to injection of allogeneic blood-derived psoriatic immunocytes: Detection of T cells expressing receptors typically present on natural killer cells, including CD94, CD158, and CD161. *Archives of Dermatology* **135**: 546–552.

[70] Krueger JG, Bowcock A (2005). Psoriasis pathophysiology: Current concepts of pathogenesis. *Annals of the Rheumatic Diseases* **64**: 30–36.

[71] Aggarwal S, Ghilardi N, Xie MH, *et al.* (2003). Interleukin-23 promotes a distinct CD4 T cell activation state characterized by the production of interleukin-17. *Journal of Biological Chemistry*; **278**: 1910–1914.

[72] Teunissen MB, Koomen CW, de Waal Malefyt R, *et al.* (1998). Interleukin-17 and interferon-g synergize in the enhancement of proinflammatory cytokine production by human keratinocytes. *Journal of Investigative Dermatology* **111**: 645–649.

[73] Nickoloff BJ (2007). Cracking the cytokine code in psoriasis. *Nature Medicine* **13**: 242–244.

[74] Kapsenberg ML, Jansen HM (2003). Antigen presentation and immunoregulation. In: *Middleton's Allergy: Principles and Practice*, 6th edn. N Franklin Adkinson Jr, JW Yunginger, WW Busse, *et al.* (eds). Mosby, St Louis, pp. 177–188.

[75] Koga T, Duan H, Urabe K, Furue M (2002). *In situ* localization of CD-38-positive dendritic cells in psoriatic lesions. *Dermatology* **204**: 100–103.

[76] Nestle FO, Turka LA, Nickoloff BJ (1994). Characterization of dermal dendritic cells in psoriasis. Autostimulation of T lymphocytes and induction of Th 1 type cytokines. *Journal of Clinical Investigation* **94**: 202–209.

[77] McGregor MJ, Barker JN, Ross EL, MacDonald DM (1992). Epidermal dendritic cells in psoriasis possess a phenotype associated with antigen presentation: *In situ* expression of beta-2 integrins. *Journal of the American Academy of Dermatology* **27**: 383–388.

[78] Cumberbatch M, Singh M, Dearman RJ, *et al.* (2006). Impaired Langerhans cell migration in psoriasis. *Journal of Experimental Medicine* **203**: 953–960.

[79] Baadsgaard O, Gupta AK, Taylor RS, *et al.* (1989). Psoriatic epidermal cells demonstrate increased numbers and function of non-Langerhans antigen presenting cells. *Journal of Investigative Dermatology* **92**: 190–195.

[80] Lowes MA, Bowcock AM, Krueger JG (2007). Pathogenesis and therapy of psoriasis. *Nature* **445**: 866–873.

[81] Deguchi M, Aiba S, Ohtani H, *et al.* (2002). Comparison of the distribution and numbers of antigen-presenting cells among T-lymphocyte-mediated dermatoses: CD1a+, factor XIIIa+, and CD68+ cells in eczematous dermatitis, psoriasis, lichen planus and graft-versus-host disease. *Archives of Dermatological Research* **294**: 297–302.

[82] Lowes MA, Chamian F, Abello MV, *et al.* (2005). Increase in TNF-a and inducible nitric oxide synthase-expressing dendritic cells in psoriasis and reduction with efalizumab (anti-CD11a). *Proceedings of the National Academy of Sciences of the United States of America* **102**: 19057–19062.

[83] Wang F, Lee E, Lowes MA, *et al.* (2006). Prominent production of IL-20 by CD68+/CD11c+ myeloid-derived cells in psoriasis: gene regulation and cellular effects. *Journal of Investigative Dermatology* **126**: 1590–1599.

[84] Wollenberg A, Wagner M, Gunther S, *et al.* (2002). Plasmacytoid dendritic cells: A new cutaneous dendritic cell subset with distinct role in inflammatory skin diseases. *Journal of Investigative Dermatology* **119**: 1096–1102.

[85] Gilliet M, Conrad C, Geiges M, *et al.* (2004). Psoriasis triggered by Toll-like receptor 7 agonist imiquimod in the presence of dermal plasmacytoid dendritic cell precursors. *Archives of Dermatology* **140**: 1490–1495.

[86] Lande R, Gregoria J, Facchinetti V, *et al.* (2007). Plasmacytoid dendritic cells sense self-DNA coupled with antimicrobial peptide. *Nature* **449**: 564–569.

[87] Nickoloff BJ (1991). The cytokine network in psoriasis. *Archives of Dermatology* **127**: 871–874.

[88] Beutler B, Cerami A (1989). The biology of cachectin/TNF: A primary mediator of the host response. *Annual Review of Immunology* **7**: 625.

[89] Borrish L, Rosenwasser LJ (2008). Cytokine production by antigen presenting cells. In: *Middleton's Allergy: Principles and Practice*, 7th edn. N Franklin Adkinson Jr, JW Yunginger, WW Busse, *et al.* (eds). Mosby, St Louis, pp. 166–168.

[90] Krueger JG (2002). The immunologic basis for the treatment of psoriasis with new biologic agents. *Journal of the American Academy of Dermatology* **46**: 1–23.

[91] Buchler T, Hajek R, Kovarova L, *et al.* (2003). Generation of antigen-loaded dendritic cells in a serum-free medium using different cytokine combinations. *Vaccine* **21**: 877–882.

[92] Ettehadi P, Greaves MW, Wallach D (1994). Elevated tumor necrosis factor-alpha biological activity in psoriatic skin lesions. *Clinical and Experimental Immunology* **96**: 146–151.

[93] Seifert M, Sterry W, Effenberger E, *et al.* (2000). The antipsoriatic activity of IL-10 is rather caused by effects on peripheral blood cells than by a direct effect on human keratinocytes. *Archives of Dermatological Research* **292**: 164–172.

[94] Asadullah K, Eskdale J, Wiese A, *et al.* (2001). Interleukin-10 promoter polymorphism in psoriasis. *Journal of Investigative Dermatology* **116**: 975–978.

[95] Menter AM, Griffiths CEM (2007). Current and future management of psoriasis. *Lancet* **370**: 272–284.

[96] Gillitzer R, Berger R, Mielke V, Muller C (1991). Upper keratinocytes of psoriatic skin lesions express high levels of NAP-1/IL-8 mRNA *in situ*. *Journal of Investigative Dermatology* **97**: 73–79.

[97] Banno T, Adachi M, Mukkamala L, Blumenberg M (2003). Unique keratinocyte-specific effects of interferon-γ that protect skin from viruses, identified using transcriptional profiling. *Antiviral Therapy* **8**: 541–554.

[98] Lew W, Bowcock AM, Krueger JG (2004). Psoriasis vulgaris: Cutaneous lymphoid tissue supports T-cell activation and 'type 1' inflammatory gene expression. *Trends in Immunology* **25**: 295–305.

[99] Gerosa F, Paganin C, Peritt D, *et al.* (1996). Interleukin-12 primes human CD4 and CD8 T cell clones for high production of both interferon-γ and interleukin-10. *Journal of Experimental Medicine* **183**: 2559–2569.

[100] Chan JR, Blumenschein W, Murphy E, *et al.* (2006). IL-23 stimulated epidermal hyperplasia via TNF and IL-20R2-dependent mechanisms with implications for psoriasis pathogenesis. *Journal of Experimental Medicine* **12**: 2577–2587.

[101] Sano S, Chan KS, Carbajal S, *et al.* (2005). Stat3 links activated keratinocytes and immunocytes required for the development of psoriasis in a novel transgenic mouse model. *Nature Medicine* **1**: 43–49.

Further reading

Farber EM (1981). Historical commentary. *Psoriasis: Proceedings of the Third International Symposium*. Grune & Stratton, New York.

Chapter 2

[1] Griffiths CEM, Christophers E, Barker JN, *et al.* (2007). A classification of psoriasis vulgaris according to phenotype. *British Journal of Dermatology* **156**: 258–262.

[2] Griffiths CEM, Camp RDR, Barker JNWN. Psoriasis. In: *Rook's Textbook of Dermatology*, 7th end. DA Burns, SM Breathnach, NH Cox, CEM Griffiths (eds). Blackwell Science, Oxford, pp. 35.1–35.69.

[3] Goodfield M, Hull SM, Holland D, *et al.* (1994). Investigations of the 'active' edge of plaque psoriasis: Vascular proliferation precedes changes in epidermal keratin. *British Journal of Dermatology* **131**: 808–813.

[4] Hagforsen E, Mustafa A, Lefvert A-K, Nordlind G (2002). Palmoplantar pustulosis: An autoimmune disease precipitated by smoking? *Acta Dermato-venereologica* **82**: 341–346.

[5] Asumalahta K, Ameen M, Suomela S, *et al.* (2003). Genetic analysis of PSORS1 distinguishes guttate psoriasis and palmoplantar pustulosis. *Journal of Investigative Dermatology* **120**: 627–632.

[6] Baker H, Ryan TJ (1968). Generalized pustular psoriasis. A clinical and epidemiological study of 104 cases. *British Journal of Dermatology* **80**: 771–793.

[7] Mease P, Goffe BS (2005). Diagnosis and treatment of psoriatic arthritis. *Journal of the American Academy of Dermatology* **52**: 1–19.

[8] Jiaravuthisan MM, Sasseville D, Vender RB, *et al.* (2007). Psoriasis of the nail: Anatomy, pathology, clinical presentation and review. *Journal of the American Academy of Dermatology* **57**: 1–27.

[9] Eastmond CJ, Wright V (1979). The nail dystrophy of psoriatic arthritis. *Annals of the Rheumatic Diseases* **38**: 226–228.

[10] Krueger GG, Callis KP (2003). Development and the use of alefacept to treat psoriasis. *Journal of the American Academy of Dermatology* **49** (Suppl.): S87–S97.

[11] Leonardi CL, Powers JL, Matheson RT, *et al.* (2003). Etanercept as monotherapy in patients with psoriasis. *New England Journal of Medicine* **349**: 2014–2022.

[12] Mease PJ, Goeffe BS, Metz J, *et al.* (2000). Etanercept in the treatment of psoriatic arthritis and psoriasis: A randomized trial. *Lancet* **356**: 385–390.

[13] Carlin CS, Feldman SR, Krueger JF, *et al.* (2004). A 50% reduction in the Psoriasis Area and Severity Index (PASI 50) is a clinically significant end point in the assessment of psoriasis. *Journal of the American Academy of Dermatology* **50**: 859–866.

Chapter 3

[1] Menter MA (1997). Psoriasis in primary care: Diagnosis and management. *Family Practice Recertification* **19**: 1–36.

[2] Roth HL (1987). Atopic dermatitis revisited. *International Journal of Dermatology* **26**: 139–149.

[3] Hanifin JM, Rajka G (1980). Diagnostic features of atopic dermatitis. *Acta Dermato-venereologica* **92** (Suppl.): 44–47.

[4] Hanifin JM, Lobitz WC Jr (1977). Newer concepts of atopic dermatitis. *Archives of Dermatology* **113**: 663.

[5] Habif TP (ed.) (2004). *Clinical Dermatology*, 4th edn. Mosby, St Louis.

[6] Devergie A (1857). Pityriasis pilaris. In: *Traite Pratique des Maladies de la Peau*, 2nd edn. Marinet, Paris, pp. 454–464.

[7] Wood GS, Reizner G (2003). Other papulusquamous disorders. In: *Dermatology*. JL Bolognia, JL Jorizzo, RP Rapini (eds). Mosby, St Louis, pp. 158–160.

[8] Wolff K, Johnson RA, Suurmond R (2005). *Fitzpatrick's Color Atlas and Synopsis of Clinical Dermatology*, 5th edn. McGraw-Hill, New York.

[9] Kossard S, Rosen R (1992). Cutaneous Bowen's disease. An analysis of 1001 cases according to age, sex, and site. *Journal of the American Academy of Dermatologists* **27**: 406.

Chapter 4

[1] Gladman DD (1995). Psoriatic arthritis. *Baillières Clinical Rheumatology* **9**: 319–329.

[2] Gladman DD, Antoni C, Mease P, *et al.* (2005). Psoriatic arthritis: Epidemiology, clinical features, course, and outcome. *Annals of the Rheumatic Diseases* **64**: 14–17.

[3] Crafford LJ (2001). Psoriatic arthritis. In: *Primer on Rheumatic Diseases*, 12th edn. JH Kippel (ed.). Arthritis Foundation, Atlanta, GA, pp. 234–238.

[4] Kammer GM, Soter NA, Gibson DJ, Schur PH (1970). Psoriatic arthritis: A clinical, immunological and HLA study of 100 patients. *Seminars in Arthritis and Rheumatism* **9**: 75–97.

[5] Mease P, Goffe BS (2005). Diagnosis and treatment of psoriatic arthritis. *Journal of the American Academy of Dermatology* **52**: 1–19.

[6] Leonard DG, O'Duffy JD, Rogers RS (1978). Prospective analysis of psoriatic arthritis in patients hospitalized for psoriasis. *Mayo Clinic Proceedings* **53**: 511–518.

[7] Gladman DD (1998). Psoriatic arthritis. *Rheumatic Diseases Clinics of North America* **24**: 829–844.

[8] Taylor WJ, Helliwell PS (2000). Case definition of psoriatic arthritis (letter). *Lancet* **356**: 2095.

[9] Zachariae H (2003). Prevalence of joint disease in patients with psoriasis: implications for therapy. *American Journal of Clinical Dermatology* **4**: 441–447.

[10] Gisondi P, Girolomoni G, Sampogna F, *et al.* (2005). Prevalence of psoriatic arthritis and joint complaints in a large population of Italian patients hospitalised for psoriasis. *European Journal of Dermatology* **15**: 279–283.

[11] Jajic Z, el Assadi G (2003). Prevalance of psoriatic arthritis in a population of patients with psoriasis. *Acta Medica Croatica* **57**: 323–326.

[12] Saraux A, Guillemin F, Guggenbul P, *et al.* (2005). Prevalence of spondyloarthropathies in France: 2001. *Annals of the Rheumatic Diseases* **64**: 1431–1435.

[13] Madland TM, Apalset EM, Johannessen AE, *et al.* (2005). Prevalence, disease manifestations, and treatment of psoriatic arthritis in Western Norway. *Journal of Rheumatology* **32**: 1918–1922.

[14] Savolainen E, Kaipianen-Seppanene O, Kroger L, Luosujarvi R (2003). Total incidence and distribution of inflammatory joint disease in a defined population: Results from the Kuopio arthritis survey. *Journal of Rheumatology* **30**: 2460–2468.

[15] Gelfand JM, Gladman DD, Mease PJ, *et al.* (2005). Epidemiology of psoriatic arthritis in the population in the United States. *Journal of the American Academy of Dermatology* **53**: 573–577.

[16] Shbeeb M, Uramoto KM, Gibson LE, *et al.* (2000). The epidemiology of psoriatic arthritis in Olmsted County, Minnesota, USA, 1982–1991. *Journal of Rheumatology* **27**: 1105–1106.

[17] Gladman DD, Shuckett R, Russell ML, *et al.* (1987). Psoriatic arthritis (PSA) – an analysis of 220 patients. *Quarterly Journal of Medicine* **62**: 127–141.

[18] Cervini C, Leardini G, Mathieu A, *et al.* (2005). Psoriatic arthritis: Epidemiology and clinical aspects in a cohort of 1,306 Italian patients. *Reumatismo* **57**: 283–290.

[19] Ruderman E, Tambar S (2004). Psoriatic arthritis: Prevalence, diagnosis, and review of therapy for the dermatologist. *Dermatologic Clinics* **22**: 477–486.

[20] Moll JM, Wright V (1973). Familial occurrence of psoriatic arthritis. *Annals of the Rheumatic Diseases* **32**: 181–201.

[21] Bowcock AM, Cookson WO (2004). The genetics of psoriasis, psoriatic arthritis and atopic dermatitis. *Human Molecular Genetics* **13** (Suppl. 1): R43.

[22] Gladman DD, Anhorn KA, Schachter RK, Mervant H (1986). HLA antigens in psoriatic arthritis. *Journal of Rheumatology* **13**: 586–592.

[23] McHugh NJ, Laurent MR, Treadwell BL, *et al.* (1987). Psoriatic arthritis: Clinical subgroups and histocompatibility antigens. *Annals of the Rheumatic Diseases* **46**: 184–188.

[24] Gladman DD, Cheung C, Ng CM, Wade JA (1999). HLA-C locus alleles in patients with psoriatic arthritis (PsA). *Human Immunology* **60**: 259–261.

[25] Liu Y, Helms C, Liao W, *et al.* (2008). A genome-wide association study of psoriasis and psoriatic arthritis identifies new disease loci. *PLoS Genetics* **4**: 1–14.

[26] Burden AD, Javed S, Bailey M, *et al.* (1998). Genetics of psoriasis: Paternal inheritance and a locus on chromosome 6p. *Journal of Investigative Dermatology* **110**: 958–960.

[27] Samuelsson L, Enlund F, Torinsson A, *et al.* (1999). A genome-wide search for genes predisposing to familial psoriasis by using a stratification approach. *Human Genetics* **105**: 523–529.

[28] Bowcock AM (1995). Genetic locus for psoriasis identified. *Annals of Medicine* **27**: 183–186.

[29] Fyrand O, Mellbye OJ, Natvig JF (1977). Immunofluorescence studies for immunoglobulins and complement C3 in synovial joint membranes in psoriatic arthritis. *Clinical and Experimental Immunology* **29**: 422–427.

[30] Costello P, Breshnihan B, O'Farrelly C, Fitzgerald O (1999). Predominance of CD8+ T lymphocytes in psoriatic arthritis. *Journal of Rheumatology* **26**: 1117–1124.

[31] Taylor WJ, Gladman DD, Helliwell PS, *et al.* (2006). Classification criteria for psoriatic arthritis: Development of new criteria from a large international study. *Arthritis and Rheumatism* **54**: 2665–2673.

[32] Harris ED Jr, Budd RC, Firestein GS, *et al.* (eds) (2005). *Harris: Kelley's Textbook of Rheumatology*, 7th edn. WB Saunders, Philadelphia.

[33] Eastmond CJ, Wright V (1979). The nail dystrophy of psoriatic arthritis. *Annals of the Rheumatic Diseases* **38**: 226–228.

[34] Helliwell PS, Hickling P, Wright V (1998). Do radiological changes of classic ankylosing spondylitis differ from the changes found in the spondylitis associated with inflammatory bowel disease, psoriasis, and reactive arthritis? *Annals of the Rheumatic Diseases* **57**: 135–140.

[35] Offidani A, Cellini A, Valeri G, Giovagnoni A (1998). Subclinical joint involvement in psoriasis: Magnetic resonance imaging and X-ray findings. *Acta Dermato-venereologica* **78**: 463–465.

[36] Kane DJ, Saxane T, Doran JP, *et al.* (2003). A comparison of ESR, CRP, serum amyloid A and cartilage oligometric matrix protein in assessing inflammation and predicting radiological outcome in early psoriatic arthritis. *Arthritis and Rheumatism* **48**: S178 (Abstr. 367).

[37] Wong K, Gladman DD, Husted J, *et al.* (1997). Mortality studies in psoriatic arthritis: Results from a single outpatient clinic. I. Causes and risk of death. *Arthritis and Rheumatism* **40**: 1868–1872.

[38] Moll JM, Wright V (1973). Psoriatic arthritis. *Seminars in Arthritis and Rheumatism* **3**: 55–78.

[39] McHugh NJ, Balachrishnan C, Jones SM (2003). Progression of peripheral joint disease in psoriatic arthritis: 5-yr prospective study. *Rheumatology* **42**: 778–783.

[40] Vasey F, Espinoza IR (1984). Psoriatic arthopathy. In: *Spondyloarthropathies*. A Calin (ed.). Grune & Straton, Orlando, FL, pp. 151–185.

[41] McGonagle D, Conaghan PG, Eincry P (1999). Psoriatic arthritis: A unified concept twenty years on. *Arthritis and Rheumatism* **42**: 1080–1086.

[42] Bennett RM (1979). Psoriatic arthritis. In: *Arthritis and Allied Conditions*, 9th edn. DJ McCarty (ed.). Lea & Febiger, Philadelphia, p. 645.

[43] Duogados M, van der Linden S, Juhlin R, *et al.* and the European Spondyloarthropathy Study Group (1991). The European Spondyloarthropathy Study Group preliminary criteria for the classification of spondyloarthropathy. *Arthritis and Rheumatism* **34**: 1218–1227.

[44] Neimann AL, Shin DB, Wang X, *et al.* (2006). Prevalence of cardiovascular risk factors in patients with psoriasis. *Journal of the American Academy of Dermatology* **55**: 829–835.

[45] Gladman DD, Farewell VT, Nadeau C (1995). Clinical indicators of progression in psoriatic arthritis: Multivariate relative risk model. *Journal of Rheumatology* **22**: 675–679.

Chapter 5

[1] Fortune DG, Richards HL, Kirby B, *et al.* (2002). A cognitive-behavioural symptom management programme as an adjunct in psoriasis therapy. *British Journal of Dermatology* **1406**: 458–465.

[2] Cornell RC, Stoughton RB (1985). Correlation of the vasoconstriction assay and clinical activity in psoriasis. *Archives of Dermatology* **121**: 63–67.

[3] van de Kerkhof PCM, Kragballe K (2005). Recommendations for the topical treatment of psoriasis. *Journal of the European Academy of Dermatology and Venereology* **19**: 495–499.

[4] Mason J, Mason AR, Cork MF (2002). Topical preparations for treatment of psoriasis: a systematic review. *British Journal of Dermatology* **146**: 351–364.

[5] Ashcroft DM, Po AL, Williams HC, Griffiths CEM (2000). Systematic review of comparative efficacy and tolerability of calcipotriol in treating chronic plaque psoriasis. *British Medical Journal* **320**: 963–967.

[6] Kragballe K, Austad J, Barnes L, *et al.* (2006). A 52-week randomised safety study of a calcipotriol/betamethasone dipropionate two-compound product (Dovobet/Daivobet/Taclonex) in the treatment of psoriasis vulgaris. *British Journal of Dermatology* **154**: 1155–1160.

[7] Gribetz C, Ling M, Lebwohl M, *et al.* (2004). Pimecrolimus cream 1% in the treatment of inter-triginous psoriasis: A double-blind, randomized study. *Journal of the American Academy of Dermatology* **51**: 731–738.

[8] Lebwohl M, Freeman AK, Chapman MS, *et al.*, Tacrolimus Ointment Study Group (2004). Tacrolimus ointment is effective for facial and intertriginous psoriasis. *Journal of the American Academy of Dermatology* **51**: 723–730.

[9] Lebwohl JG, Breneman DL, Goffe BS, *et al.* (1998). Tazarotene 0.1% gel plus corticosteroid cream in the treatment of plaque psoriasis. *Journal of the American Academy of Dermatology* **39**: 590–596.

[10] Goeckerman WH (1925). Treatment of psoriasis. *Northwest Medicine* **24**: 229–231.

[11] Ingram JT (1953). The approach to psoriasis. *British Medical Journal* **2**: 591–594.

[12] British Photodermatology Group (1997). An appraisal of narrowband (TL-01) UV-B phototherapy. British Photodermatology Group. *British Journal of Dermatology* **137**: 327–330.

[13] Nguyen T, Young M, Menter A (1997). UVB phototherapy for psoriasis. *Dermatologic Therapy* **4**: 11–23.

[14] Parrish JA, Jaenicke KF (1981). Action spectrum for phototherapy of psoriasis. *Journal of Investigative Dermatology* **76**: 359–362.

[15] Coven TR, Burack LH, Gilleaudeau R, *et al.* (1997). Narrowband UV-B produces superior clinical and histopathological resolution of moderate-to-severe psoriasis in patients compared with broadband UV-B. *Archives of Dermatology* **133**: 1514–1522.

[16] Tanew A, Radakovic-Fijan S, Schemper M, Honigsmann H (1999). Narrowband UV-B phototherapy vs. photochemotherapy in the treatment of chronic plaque-type psoriasis: A paired comparison study. *Archives of Dermatology* **135**: 519–524.

[17] Gibbs NK, Traynor JN, MacKie RM, *et al.* (1995). The phototumorigenic potential of broad-band (270–350 nm) and narrow-band (311–313 nm) phototherapy sources cannot be predicted by their edematogenic potential in hairless mouse skin. *Journal of Investigative Dermatology* **104**: 359–363.

[18] Gordon PM, Diffey BL, Matthews JNS, Farr PM (1999). A randomized comparison of narrowband TL-01 phototherapy and PUVA photochemotherapy for psoriasis. *Journal of the American Academy of Dermatology* **41**: 728–732.

[19] Morison WL (2003). Systemic and topical PUVA therapy. In: *Therapy of Moderate-to-Severe Psoriasis*. GD Weinstein, AB Gottlieb (eds). Marcel Dekker, New York, pp. 53–90.

[20] Menter A, Cram DL (1983). The Goeckerman regimen in two psoriasis day care centers. *Journal of the American Academy of Dermatology* **9**: 59–65.

[21] Kemeny L, Bonis B, Dobozy A, *et al.* (2001). 308-nm excimer laser therapy for psoriasis. *Archives of Dermatology* **137**: 95–96.

[22] Taibjee SM, Cheung ST, Laube S, Lanigan SW (2005). Controlled study of excimer and pulsed dye lasers in the treatment of psoriasis. *British Journal of Dermatology* **153**: 960–966.

[23] Parrish JA, Fitzpatrick TB, Tanenbaum L, Pathak MA (1974). Photochemotherapy of psoriasis with oral methoxsalen and longwave ultraviolet. *New England Journal of Medicine* **291**: 1207–1211.

[24] Melski JW, Tanenbaum L, Parrish JA, *et al.*, and 28 participating investigators (1977). Oral methoxsalen photochemotherapy for the treatment of psoriasis: A cooperative clinical trial. *Journal of Investigative Dermatology* **68**: 328–335.

[25] Stern RS, Lange R (1988). Non-melanoma skin cancer occurring in patients treated with PUVA five to ten years after first treatment. *Journal of Investigative Dermatology* **91**: 120–124.

[26] Stern RS (2001). PUVA follow up group. The risk of melanoma in association with long-term exposure to PUVA. *Journal of the American Academy of Dermatology* **44**: 755–761.

[27] Grundmann-Kollmann M, Ludwig R, Zollner TM, *et al.* (2004). Narrowband UVB and cream psoralen-UVA combination therapy for plaque-type psoriasis. *Journal of the American Academy of Dermatology* **50**: 734–739.

[28] Turner RJ, Walshaw D, Diffey BL, Farr PM (2000). A controlled study of ultraviolet A sunbed treatment of psoriasis. *British Journal of Dermatology* **143**: 957–963.

[29] Krueger G, Koo J, Lebwohl M, *et al.* (2001). The impact of psoriasis on quality of life. Results of a 1998 National Psoriasis Foundation patient membership survey. *Archives of Dermatology* **137**: 280–284.

[30] Liem WH, McCollough JL, Weinstein GD (1995). Effectiveness of topical therapy for psoriasis: Results of a national survey. *Cutis* **55**: 306–310.

[31] Heydendael VM, Spuls PI, Opmeer BC, *et al.* (2003). Methotrexate versus ciclosporine in moderate-to-severe chronic plaque psoriasis. *New England Journal of Medicine* **349**: 658–665.

[32] Menter A, Korman N, Elmets C, *et al.* (2009). Management of psoriasis and psoriatic arthritis: Section 4: Guidelines of care for the management and treatment of psoriasis with traditional systemic agents. *Journal of the American Academy of Dermatology* **61**(3):451–485.

[33] Boffa MJ, Smith A, Chalmers RJG, *et al.* (1996). Serum type III procollagen aminopeptide for assessing liver damage in methotrexate-treated psoriatic patients. *British Journal of Dermatology* **135**: 538–544.

[34] Zachariae H, Aslam HM, Bjerring P, *et al.* (1991). Serum aminoterminal propeptide of type III pro-collagen in psoriasis and psoriatic arthritis: Relation to liver fibrosis and arthritis. *Journal of the American Academy of Dermatology* **25**: 50–53.

[35] Roenigk HH Jr, Auerbach R, Maibach H, *et al.* (1998). Methotrexate in psoriasis: Consensus conference. *Journal of the American Academy of Dermatology* **38**: 478–485.

[36] Mueller W, Hermann B (1979). Ciclosporin for psoriasis. *New England Journal of Medicine* **301**: 555.

[37] Ellis CN, Fradin MS, Messana JM, *et al.* (1991). Cyclosporine for plaque-type psoriasis: Results of a multi-dose, double-blind trial. *New England Journal of Medicine* **324**: 277–284.

[38] Finzi AF (ed.) (1993). *Cyclosporin in severe psoriasis: The Italian experience (Dermatology).* S Karger, Basel.

[39] Berth-Jones J, Henderson CA, Munro CS, *et al.* (1997). Treatment of psoriasis with intermittent short-course cyclosporin (Neoral). A multicentre study. *British Journal of Dermatology* **136**: 527–530.

[40] Ho VCY, Albrecht G, Vanaclocha F, *et al.* (1999). Intermittent short courses of cyclosporin (Neoral) for psoriasis unresponsive to topical therapy: A 1-year multicentre, randomised study. *British Journal of Dermatology* **141**: 283–291.

[41] Griffiths CEM, Dubertret L, Ellis CH, *et al.* (2004). Ciclosporin in psoriasis clinical practice: an international consensus statement. *British Journal of Dermatology* **150** (Suppl. 67): 11–23.

[42] Paul CF, Ho VC, McGeown C, *et al.* (2003). Risk of malignancies in psoriasis treated with ciclosporin: A 5-yr cohort study. *Journal of Investigative Dermatology* **120**: 211–216.

[43] Gollnick HP, Dummler U (1997). Retinoids. *Clinical Dermatology* **15**: 799–810.

[44] Nijsten TE, Stern RS (2003). Oral retinoid use reduces cutaneous squamous cell carcinoma risk in patients with psoriasis treated with psoralen-UVA: A nested cohort study. *Journal of the American Academy of Dermatology* **49**: 644–650.

[45] Connetics Corporation (2004). Soriatane (acitretin) capsules. Complete product information.

[46] Koo J (1999). Systemic sequential therapy of psoriasis: A new paradigm for improved therapeutic results. *Journal of the American Academy of Dermatology* **41**: S25–S28.

[47] Mroweitz U, Christophers E, Altmeyer P (1999). Treatment of severe psoriasis with fumaric acid esters: Scientific background and guidelines for therapeutic use. The German Fumaric Acid Ester Consensus Conference. *British Journal of Dermatology* **141**: 424–429.

[48] Fumedica Pharmaceuticals (2003). Fumaderm. Summary of product characteristics.

[49] Gollnick H, Altmeyer P, Kaufmann R, *et al.* (2002). Topical calcipotriol plus oral fumaric acid is more effective and faster acting than oral fumaric acid monotherapy in the treatment of severe chronic plaque psoriasis vulgaris. *Dermatology* **205**: 46–53.

[50] Mrowietz U, Altmeyer P, Bieber T, *et al.* (2007). Treatment of psoriasis with fumaric acid esters (Fumaderm). *Journal der Deutschen Dermatologischen Gesellschaft* **5**: 716–717.

[51] Menter MA, Krueger GC, Feldman SR, Weinstein GD (2003). Psoriasis treatment 2003 at the new millennium: Position paper on behalf of the authors. *Journal of the American Academy of Dermatology* **49**: S39–S43.

[52] Krueger JG (2002). The immunologic basis for the treatment of psoriasis with new biologic agents. *Journal of the American Academy of Dermatology* **46**: 1–26.

[53] Sterry W (2004). Biologicals in psoriasis consensus. *British Journal of Dermatology* **151** (Suppl. 69): 1–17.

[54] Griffiths CEM (2004). T-Cell-targeted biologicals for psoriasis. *Current Drug Targets. Inflammation and Allergy* **3**: 157–161.

[55] Lebwohl M, Christophers E, Langley R, *et al.* (2003). An international, randomized, double-blind, placebo-controlled phase 3 trial of intra-muscular alefacept in patients with chronic plaque psoriasis. *Archives of Dermatology* **139**: 719–727.

[56] Menter A, Cather JC, Baker D, *et al.* (2006). The efficacy of multiple courses of alefacept in patients with moderate to severe chronic plaque psoriasis. *Journal of the American Academy of Dermatology* **54**: 61–63.

[57] Perlmutter A, Cather J, Franks B, *et al.* (2008). Alefacept revisited: Our 3-year clinical experience in 200 patients with chronic plaque psoriasis. *Journal of the American Academy of Dermatology* **58**: 116–124.

[58] Papp KA, Bissonnette R, Krueger JG, *et al.* (2001). The treatment of moderate to severe psoriasis with a new anti-CD11a monoclonal antibody. *Journal of the American Academy of Dermatology* **45**: 665–674.

[59] Gottlieb AB, Hamilton T, Caro I, *et al.* (2006). Long-term continuous efalizumab therapy in patients with moderate to severe chronic plaque psoriasis: Updated results from an ongoing trial. *Journal of the American Academy of Dermatology* **54**: S154–S163.

[60] Leonardi C, Menter A, Hamilton T, *et al* (2008). Efalizumab: results of a 3-year continuous dosing study for the long-term control of psoriasis. *British Journal of Dermatology* **158**: 1107–1116.

[61] Mease PJ, Goffe BS, Metz J, *et al.* (2000). Etanercept in the treatment of psoriatic arthritis and psoriasis: A randomised trial. *Lancet* **356**: 385–390.

[62] Leonardi CL, Powers JL, Matheson RT, *et al.* (2003). Etanercept as monotherapy in patients with psoriasis. *Journal of the American Academy of Dermatology* **349**: 2014–2022.

[63] Tyring S, Gottlieb A, Papp K, *et al.* (2006). Etanercept and clinical outcomes, fatigue, and depression: Double-blind placebo-controlled ran-domised phase III trial. *Lancet* **367**: 29–35.

[64] Krueger GG, Langley RG, Finlay AY, *et al.* (2005). Patient-reported outcomes of psoriasis improve-ment with etanercept therapy: Results of a ran-domized phase III trial. *British Journal of Dermatology* **153**: 1192–1199.

[65] Mease PJ, Kivitz AJ, Burch FX, *et al.* (2004). Etanercept treatment of psoriatic arthritis. *Arthritis and Rheumatism* **50**: 2264–2272.

[66] Paller AS, Siegfried EC, Langley RG, *et al.* (2008). Etanercept treatment for children and adolescents with plaque psoriasis. *New England Journal of Medicine* **358**: 241–251.

[67] Gordon KB, Langley RG, Leonardi C, *et al.* (2006). Clinical response to adalimumab treatment in patients with moderate to severe psoriasis: Double-blind, randomized controlled trial and open-label extension study. *Journal of the American Academy of Dermatology* **55**: 598–606.

[68] Menter A, Tyring SK, Gordon K, *et al.* (2008). Adalimumab therapy for moderate to severe psoriasis: A randomized, controlled phase III trial. *Journal of the American Academy of Dermatology* **58**: 106–115.

[69] Winterfield L, Menter A (2004). Psoriasis and its treatment with infliximab-mediated tumor necrosis factor α blockade. *Dermatologic Clinics* **22**: 437–447.

[70] Reich K, Nestle FO, Papp K, *et al.* (2005). Infliximab induction and maintenance therapy for moderate-to-severe psoriasis: A phase III, multi-centre, double-blind trial. *Lancet* **366**: 1367–1374.

[71] Menter A, Feldman SR, Weinstein GD, *et al.* (2007). A randomized comparison of continuous vs. intermittent infliximab maintenance regimens over 1 year in the treatment of moderate-to-severe plaque psoriasis. *Journal of the American Academy of Dermatology* **56**: 31.e1–31.e15.

[72] Feldman SR, Gordon KB, Bala M, *et al.* (2005). Infliximab treatment results in significant improvement in the quality of life of patients with severe psoriasis: A double-blind placebo-controlled trial. *British Journal of Dermatology* **152**: 954–960.

[73] Antoni C, Krueger GG, de Vlam K, *et al.* (2005). Infliximab improves signs and symptoms of psoriatic arthritis: Results of the IMPACT 2 trial. *Annals of the Rheumatic Diseases* **64**: 1150–1157.

[74] Smith CH, Anstey AV, Barker JN, *et al.* (2005). British Association of Dermatologists Guidelines for the use of biological interventions in psoriasis 2005. *British Journal of Dermatology* **153**: 486–497.

[75] Rosemarin D, Strober B (2005). The potential of interlukin 12 inhibition in the treatment of psoriasis. *Journal of Drugs in Dermatology* 4: 318–325.

[76] Menter AM, Griffiths CEM (2007). Current and future management of psoriasis. *Lancet* **370**: 272–284.

[77] van de Kerkhof PCM (2003). Psoriasis. In: *Dermatology*. JL Bolognia, JL Jorizzo, RP Rapini (eds). Mosby, St Louis, pp. 125–149.

[78] Yawalkar N, Karlen S, Hunger R, et al. (1998). Expression of interleukin-12 is increased in psoriatic skin. *Journal of Investigative Dermatology* **111**: 1053–1057.

[79] Harrington LE, Hatton RD, Mangan PR, et al. (2005). Interleukin 17-producing CD4+ effector T cells develop via a lineage distinct from the T helper type 1 and 2 lineages. *Nature Immunology* **6**: 1123–1132.

[80] Park H, Li Z, Yang XO, et al. (2005). A distinct lineage of CD4 T cells regulates tissue inflammation by producing interleukin 17. *Nature Immunology* **6**: 1133–1141.

[81] Lowes MA, Lew W, Krueger JG (2004). Current concepts in the immunopathogenesis of psoriasis. *Dermatologic Clinics* **22**: 349–369.

[82] Cargill M, Schrodi SJ, Chang M, et al. (2007). A large-scale genetic association study confirms IL12B and leads to the identification of IL23R as psoriasis-risk genes. *American Journal of Human Genetics* **80**: 273–390.

[83] Leonardi CL, Kimball AB, Papp KA, et al. (2008). Efficacy and safety of ustekinumab, a human interleukin-12/23 monoclonal antibody, in patients with psoriasis: 76-week results from a randomised, double-blind, placebo-controlled trial (PHOENIX 1). *Lancet* **371**: 1665–1674.

[84] Papp KA, Langley RG, Lebwohl M, et al. (2008). Efficacy and safety of ustekinumab, a human interleukin-12/23 monoclonal antibody, in patients with psoriasis: 52-week results from a randomised, double-blind, placebo-controlled trial (PHOENIX 2). *Lancet* **371**: 1675–1684.

[85] Gottlieb A, Menter A, Mendelsohn A, et al. (2009). Ustekinumab, a human interleukin 12/23 monoclonal antibody, for psoriatic arthritis: a randomised, double-blind, placebo-controlled, crossover trial. *Lancet* **373**: 633–640.

[86] Gordon K, Leonardi C, Lebwohl M, et al. (2009). *The ustekinumab safety experience in patients with moderate-to-severe psoriasis: Results from pooled analyses of phase 2 and phase 3 clinical trial data.* Abstract presented at the 18th Congress of the European Academy of Dermatology and Venerology.

[87] Menter MA, Abramovits W (1999). Rotational, sequential and combination regimens in the treatment of psoriasis (abstract). *Dermatologic Therapy* **11**: 88–95.

[88] Koo J (1997). Calcipotriol/calcipotriene (Dovonex/Daivonex) in combination with phototherapy: A review. *Journal of the American Academy of Dermatology* **37**: S59–S61.

[89] Grupper C, Berretti B (1981). Treatment of psoriasis by oral PUVA therapy combined with aromatic retinoid (Ro 10-9359; Tigason). *Dermatologica* **162**: 404–413.

[90] Lowe NJ, Prystowsky J, Armstrong RB (1991). Acitretin plus UVB therapy for psoriasis. *Journal of the American Academy of Dermatology* **4**: 591–594.

[91] Ruzicka T, Sommerburg C, Braun-Falco O, et al. (1990). Efficiency of acitretin in combination with UVB in the treatment of severe psoriasis. *Archives of Dermatology* **126**: 482–486.

[92] Molin L, Larko O (1997). Cancer induction by immunosuppression in psoriasis after heavy PUVA treatment (letter). *Acta Dermato-venereologica* **77**: 402.

[93] Menter MA, See JA, Amend WJC, et al. (1996). Proceedings of the Psoriasis Combination and Rotation Therapy Conference. Deer Valley, Utah, October 7–9, 1994. *Journal of the American Academy of Dermatology* **34**: 315–321.

[94] Rosenbaum MM, Roenigk HH Jr (1984). Treatment of generalized pustular psoriasis with etretinate (Ro 10-9359) and methotrexate. *Journal of the American Academy of Dermatology* **10**: 357–361.

[95] Tugwell P, Pincus T, Yocum D, et al. (1995). Combination therapy with ciclosporin and methotrexate in severe rheumatoid arthritis. *New England Journal of Medicine* **333**: 137–141.

[96] Stein CM, Pincus T, Yocum D, *et al*. (1997). Combination treatment of severe rheumatoid arthritis with ciclosporin and methotrexate for forty-eight weeks: An open-label extension study. *Arthritis and Rheumatism* **40**: 1843–1851.

[97] Clark CM, Kirby B, Morris AD, *et al*. (1999). Combination treatment with methotrexate and ciclosporin for severe recalcitrant psoriasis. *British Journal of Dermatology* **141**: 279–282.

[98] Grossman RM, Thivolet J, Claudy A, *et al*. (1994). A novel therapeutic approach to psoriasis with combination calcipotriol ointment and very low-dose cyclosporine: Results of a multicenter placebo-controlled study. *Journal of the American Academy of Dermatology* **31**: 68–74.

[99] Kirby B, Harrison PV (1999). Combination low-dose cyclosporine (Neoral) and hydroxyurea for severe recalcitrant psoriasis. *British Journal of Dermatology* **140**: 186–187.

[100] van de Kerkhof PC, Cambazard F, Hutchinson PE, *et al*. (1998). The effect of addition of calcipotriol ointment (50 micrograms/g) to acitretin therapy in psoriasis. *British Journal of Dermatology* **138**: 84–89.

[101] van der Rhee HJ, Tijssen JGP, Herrmann WA, *et al*. (1980). Combined treatment of psoriasis with a new aromatic retinoid (Tigason) in a low dosage orally and triamcinolone acetonide cream topically: A double-blind trial. *British Journal of Dermatology* **102**: 203–212.

[102] Orfanos CE, Runne U (1976). Systemic use of a new retinoid with and without local dithranol treatment in generalized psoriasis. *British Journal of Dermatology* **95**: 101–103.

[103] Polano MK, van der Rhee HJ, van der Schroeff JG (1982). A three-year follow-up study of psoriasis patients treated with low dosages of etretinate orally and corticosteroids topically. *Acta Dermato-venereologica* **62**: 361–364.

[104] Salomon D, Mesheit J, Masgrau-Peya F, *et al*. (1994). Acitretin does not prevent psoriasis relapse related to cyclosporine A tapering. *Journal of the American Academy of Dermatology* **130**: 257–258.

[105] Tuyp E, MacKie RM (1986). Combination therapy for psoriasis with methotrexate and etretinate. *Journal of the American Academy of Dermatology* **14**: 70–73.

[106] Zachariae H (1984). Methotrexate and etretinate as concurrent therapies in the treatment of psoriasis (letter). *Archives of Dermatology* **120**: 155.

[107] Beck HL, Foged EK (1983). Toxic hepatitis due to combination therapy with methotrexate and etretinate in psoriasis. *Dermatologica* **167**: 94–96.

[108] Cather JC, Menter A (2005). Combining traditional agents and biologics for the treatment of psoriasis. *Seminars in Cutaneous Medicine and Surgery* **24**: 37–45.

[109] Mease PJ, Gladman DD, Keystone EC; Alefacept in Psoriatic Arthritis Study Group (2006). Alefacept in combination with methotrexate for the treatment of psoriatic arthritis: results of a randomized, double-blind, placebo-controlled study. *Arthritis and Rheumatism* **54**: 1638–1645.

[110] Weinstein GD, White GM (1993). An approach to the treatment of moderate to severe psoriasis with rotational therapy. *Journal of the American Academy of Dermatology* **28**: 454–459.

[111] Koo J (1994). Systemic sequential therapy of psoriasis: A new paradigm for improved therapeutic results. *Journal of the American Academy of Dermatology* **41**: S25–S28.

[112] National Psoriasis Foundation. New drugs in development. Available from: *www.psoriasis.org/research/pipeline/chart.php*. Updated March 2008.

[113] Saurat JH, Stingl G, Dubertret L, *et al*. (2008). Efficacy and safety results from the randomized controlled comparative study of adalimumab vs. methotrexate vs. placebo in patients with psoriasis (CHAMPION). *British Journal of Dermatology* **158**: 558–566.

[114] Janssen-Ortho Inc. (2008). Stelara (ustekinumab) product monograph. Janssen-Ortho, Toronto, Ontario.

[115] Kimball AB, Gordon KB, Langley RG, *et al*. (2008). Safety and efficacy of ABT-874, a fully human interleukin 12/23 monoclonal antibody, in the treatment of moderate to severe chronic plaque psoriasis. *Archives of Dermatology* **144**: 200–207.

[116] Detmar M, Brown LF, Claffey KP, *et al*. (1994). Overexpression of vascular permeability factor/vascular endothelial growth factor and its receptors in psoriasis. *Journal of Experimental Medicine* **180**: 1141–1146.

[117] Creamer D, Allen MH, Groves RW, Barker JNWN (1996). Circulating vascular permeability factor/vascular endothelial growth factor erythroderma. *Lancet* **348**: 1101.

[118] Young HS, Summers AM, Bhushan M, *et al.* (2004). Single nucleotide polymorphisms of vascular endothelial growth factor (VEGF) in psoriasis of early onset. *Journal of Investigative Dermatology* **122**: 209–215.

[119] Xia Y-P, Li B, Hylton D (2003). Transgenic delivery of VEGF to mouse skin leads to an inflammatory condition resembling human psoriasis. *Blood* **102**: 161–168.

[120] Genentech Inc (2006). Avastin (bevacizumab) package insert. Genentech, South San Francisco, CA.

[121] Wilson JF (2004). Angiogenesis therapy moves beyond cancer. *Annals of Internal Medicine* **141**: 165–168.

[122] Gottlieb AB, Griffiths CE, Ho VC, *et al.* (2005). Oral pimecrolimus in the treatement of moderate to severe chronic plaque-type psoriasis: A double-blind, multicentre, randomized, dose-finding trial. *British Journal of Dermatology* **152**: 1219–1227.

[123] Bissonette R, Papp K, Poulin Y, *et al.* (2006). A randomized, multicenter, double-blind, placebo-controlled phase 2 trial of ISA247 in patients with chronic plaque type psoriasis. *Journal of the American Academy of Dermatology* **54**: 472–478.

[124] Feldman SR, Mellen BG, Housman TS, *et al.* (2002). Efficacy of the 308-nm excimer laser for treatment of psoriasis: Results of a multicenter study. *Journal of the American Academy of Dermatology* **46**: 900–906.

[125] Leeuw J, Bhupendra T, Bjerring P, *et al.* (2006). Concomitant treatment of psoriasis of the hands and feet with pulsed dye laster and topical calcipotriol, salicylic acid, or both: A prospective open study in 41 patients. *Journal of the American Academy of Dermatology* **54**: 266–271.

[126] Warren RB, Griffiths CEM (2005). The potential of pharmacogenetics in optimizing the use of methotrexate for psoriasis. *British Journal of Dermatology* **153**: 869–873.

[127] Young HS, Summers AM, Read IR, *et al.* (2006). Interaction between genetic control of vascular endothelial growth factor production and retinoid responsiveness in psoriasis. *Journal of Investigative Dermatology* **126**: 453–459.

Chapter 6

[1] Krueger G, Koo J, Lebwohl M, *et al.* (2001). The impact of psoriasis on quality of life: Results of a 1998 National Psoriasis Foundation patient membership survey. *Archives of Dermatology* **137**: 280–284.

[2] Gupta MA, Gupta AK (1998). Depression and suicidal ideation in dermatology patients with acne, alopecia arcata, atopic dermatitis, and psoriasis. *British Journal of Dermatology* **139**: 846–850.

[3] Finlay AY, Coles EC (1995). The effect of severe psoriasis on the quality of life of 369 patients. *British Journal of Dermatology* **132**: 236–244.

[4] Menter MA, Mease PJ (2006). Quality-of-life issues in psoriasis and psoriatic arthritis: Outcome measures and therapies from a dermatological perspective. *Journal of the American Academy of Dermatology* **54**: 685–704.

[5] Guyatt GH, Feeny DH, Patrick DL (1993). Measuring health-related quality of life. *Annals of Internal Medicine* **118**: 622–629.

[6] Menter A, Griffiths CE (2007). Current and future management of psoriasis. *Lancet* **370**: 272–284.

[7] De Korte J, Sprangers MA, Mombers FM, Bos JD (2004). Quality of life in patients with psoriasis: A systematic literature review. *Journal of Investigative Dermatology. Symposium Proceedings* **9**: 140–147.

[8] Rapp, SR, Feldman SR, Exum ML, *et al.* (1999). Psoriasis causes as much disability as other major medical diseases. *Journal of the American Academy of Dermatology* **41**: 401–407.

[9] Horn EJ, Fox KM, Patel V, *et al.* (2007). Association of patient-reported psoriasis severity with income and employment. *Journal of the American Academy of Dermatology* **57**: 963–971.

[10] Gupta MA, Gupta AK (1995). Age and gender differences in the impact of psoriasis on quality of life. *International Journal of Dermatology* **34**: 700–703.

[11] Feldman SR, Fleischer AB Jr, Reboussin DM, *et al.* (1997). The economic impact of psoriasis severity. *Journal of the American Academy of Dermatology* **37**: 564–569.

[12] Gupta MA, Schork NJ, Gupta AK, *et al.* (1993). Suicidal ideation in psoriasis. *International Journal of Dermatology* **32**: 188–190.

[13] McKenna KE, Stern RS (1997). The impact of psoriasis on the quality of life of patients from a 16-center PUVA follow-up cohort. *Journal of the American Academy of Dermatology* **36**: 388–394.

[14] Koo JY (1996). Population-based epidemiological study of psoriasis with emphasis on quality of life assessment. *Dermatologic Clinics* **14**: 485–496.

[15] Zachariae R, Zachariae H, Blomqvist K, *et al.* (2002). Quality of life in 6497 Nordic patients with psoriasis. *British Journal of Dermatology* **146**: 1006–1016.

[16] Esposito M, Saraceno R, Giunta A, *et al.* (2006). An Italian study on psoriasis and depression. *Dermatology* **212**: 123–127.

[17] Gupta MA, Gupta AK, Kirby S, *et al.* (1988). Pruritus in psoriasis. A prospective study of some psychiatric and dermatologic correlates. *Archives of Dermatology* **124**: 1052–1057.

[18] Devrimci-Ozguven H, Kundakci N, Kumbasar H, Boyvat A (2000). The depression, anxiety, life satisfaction and affective expression levels in psoriasis patients. *Journal of the European Academy of Dermatology and Venereology* **14**: 267–271.

[19] Griffiths CE, Richards HL (2001). Psychological influences in psoriasis. *Clinical and Experimental Dermatology* **26**: 338–342.

[20] Fortune DG, Main CJ, O'Sullivan TM, Griffiths CEM (1997). Quality of life in patients with psoriasis: The contribution of clinical variables and psoriasis-specific stress. *British Journal of Dermatology* **137**: 755–760.

[21] Mukhtar R, Choi J, Koo JY (2004). Quality-of-life issues in psoriasis. *Dermatologic Clinics* **22**: 389–395.

[22] Gupta MA, Gupta AK (1997). Psoriasis and sex: A study of moderately to severely affected patients. *International Journal of Dermatology* **36**: 259–262.

[23] Ginsburg IH, Link BG (1993). Psychological consequences of rejection and stigma feelings in psoriasis patients. *International Journal of Dermatology* **32**: 587–591.

[24] Rapp SR, Cottrell CA, Leary MR (2001). Social coping strategies associated with quality of life decrements among psoriasis patients. *British Journal of Dermatology* **145**: 610–616.

[25] Scharloo M, Kaptein AA, Weinman J (2000). Patients' illness perceptions and coping as predictors of functional status in psoriasis: A 1-year follow-up. *British Journal of Dermatology* **142**: 899–907.

[26] Jenkinson C, Coulter A, Wright L (1993). Short Form 36 (SF-36) health survey questionnaire: Normative data for adults of working age. *British Medical Journal* **306**: 1437–1440.

[27] Garratt AM, Ruta DA, Abdalla MI, *et al.* (1993). The SF-36 health survey questionnaire: An outcome measure suitable for routine clinical use within the NHS? *British Medical Journal* **306**: 1440–1444.

[28] Ware JE Jr, Snow KK, Kosinski M (2000). *SF-36 Health Survey: Manual and Interpretation Guide*. Quality Metric, Lincoln, RI.

[29] Heydendael VM, de Borgie CA, Spuls PI, *et al.* (2004). The burden of disease of psoriasis is not determined by disease severity only. *Journal of Investigative Dermatology. Symposium Proceedings* **9**: 131–135.

[30] Wallenhammer LM, Nyfjall M, Lindberg M, *et al.* (2004). Health-related quality of life and hand eczema – a comparison of two instruments, including factor analysis. *Journal of Investigative Dermatology* **122**: 1381–1389.

[31] Lewis VJ, Finaly AY (2005). A critical review of quality-of-life scales for psoriasis. *Dermatologic Clinics* **23**: 707–716.

[32] Mease PJ, Gottlieb AB, Wanke LA, Burge DJ (2003). Sustained improvement in activities of daily living and vitality in patients with psoriatic arthritis treated with etanercept. *Arthritis and Rheumatism* **46**: 9.

[33] Mease PJ, Kivitz AJ, Burch FX, *et al.* (2004). Etanercept treatment of psoriatic arthritis. Safety, efficacy, and effect on disease progression. *Arthritis and Rheumatism* **50**: 2264–2272.

[34] Fries JF, Spitz P, Kraines RG, Holman HR (1980). Measurement of patient outcome in arthritis. *Arthritis and Rheumatism* **23**: 137–145.

[35] Blackmore MG, Gladman DD, Husted J, *et al.* (1995). Measuring health status in psoriatic arthritis: The Health Assessment Questionnaire and its modification. *Journal of Rheumatology* **22**: 886–893.

[36] Finlay AY, Khan GK (1994). Dermatology Life Quality Index (DLQI): A simple practical measure for routine clinical use. *Clinical and Experimental Dermatology* **19**: 210–216.

[37] Nichol MB, Margolies JI, Lippa E, *et al.* (1996). The application of multiple quality-of-life instruments in individuals with mild-to-moderate psoriasis. *Pharmacoeconomics* **10**: 644–653.

[38] Finlay AY, Kelley SE (1987). Psoriasis – an index of disability. *Clinical and Experimental Dermatology* **12**: 8–11.

[39] Finlay AY, Coles EC (1995). The effect of severe psoriasis on the quality of life of 369 patients. *British Journal of Dermatology* **132**: 236–244.

[40] Lewis VJ, Finlay AY (2005). Two decades experience of the Psoriasis Disability Index. *Dermatology* **210**: 261–268.

[41] Finlay AY, Khan GK, Luscombe DK, Salek MS (1990). Validation of Sickness Impact Profile and Psoriasis Disability Index in psoriasis. *British Journal of Dermatology* **123**: 751–756.

[42] Root S, Kent G, al Abadie MS (1994). The relationship between disease severity, disability and psychological distress in patients undergoing PUVA treatment for psoriasis. *Dermatology* **189**: 234–237.

[43] O'Neill P, Kelly P (1996). Postal questionnaire study of disability in the community associated with psoriasis. *British Medical Journal* **313**: 919–921.

[44] Gupta G, Long J, Tillman DM (1999). The efficacy of narrowband ultraviolet B phototherapy in psoriasis using objective and subjective outcome measures. *British Journal of Dermatology* **140**: 887–890.

[45] Kirby B, Fortune DG, Bhushan M (2000). The Salford Psoriasis Index: An holistic measure of psoriasis severity. *British Journal of Dermatology* **142**: 728–732.

[46] Kirby B, Richards HL, Woo P (2001). Physical and psychologic measures are necessary to assess overall psoriasis severity. *Journal of the American Academy of Dermatology* **45**: 72–76.

[47] Koo J, Menter A (2003). The Koo–Menter instrument for identification of psoriasis patients requiring systemic therapy. *National Psoriasis Foundation Psoriasis Forum* **9**: 6–9.

[48] Feldman SR, Koo JY, Menter A, Bagel J (2005). Decision points for the initiation of systemic treatment of psoriasis. *Journal of the American Academy of Dermatology* **53**: 101–107.

[49] Koo JY, Kozma CM, Menter A, Lebwohl M (2003). *Development of a disease-specific quality of life questionnaire: The 12-item psoriasis quality of life questionnaire (PQOL-12).* Presented at the 61st Annual Meeting of the American Academy of Dermatology, San Francisco, CA.

[50] Koo JY (1996). Population-based epidemiologic study of psoriasis with emphasis on quality of life assessment. *Dermatologic Clinics* **14**: 485–496.

[51] Koo JY, Kowalski J, Guenther L, Walker P (2004). *Quality of life effect of oral tazarotene in patients with moderate to severe psoriasis as measured by 12-item psoriasis quality of life questionnaire (PQOL-12).* Presented at the 62nd Annual Meeting of the American Academy of Dermatology, Washington, DC.

[52] Felson DT, Anderson JJ, Boers M, *et al.* (1995). The American College of Rheumatology. Preliminary definition of improvement in rheumatoid arthritis. *Arthritis and Rheumatism* **38**: 727–735.

[53] Han C, Smolen JS, Kavanaugh A, *et al.* (2007). The impact of infliximab treatment on quality of life in patients with inflammatory rheumatic diseases. *Arthritis Research and Therapy* **9**: R103.

[54] Mease P, Gladman D, Ritchlin C, *et al.* (2004). Adalimumab therapy in patients with psoriatic arthritis: 24-week results of a phase III study. *Arthritis and Rheumatism* **50**: 4097.

[55] Mease PJ, Antoni CE, Gladman DD, Talylor WJ (2005). Psoriatic arthritis assessment tools in clinical trials. *Annals of Rheumatic Diseases* **64**: 49–54.

[56] McKenna SP, Doward LC, Whalley D, *et al.*
(2004). Development of the PsAQoL: A quality of
life instrument specific to psoriatic arthritis.
Annals of Rheumatic Diseases **63**: 162–169.

[57] Boers M, Brooks P, Strand CV, Tugwell P (1998).
The OMERACT filter for Outcome Measures
in Rheumatology. *Journal of Rheumatology*
25: 198–199.

[58] The Outcome Measures in Rheumatology
(OMERACT) website. Available from:
www.omeract.org.

Chapter 7

[1] Kourosh AS, Miner A, Menter A (2008). Psoriasis
as the marker of underlying systemic disease.
Skin Therapy Letter **13**: 1–5.

[2] McDonald CJ, Calabresi P (1973). Occlusive
vascular disease in psoriatic patients. *New England
Journal of Medicine* **288**: 912.

[3] Ena P, Madeddu P, Glorioso N, *et al.* (1985). High
prevalence of cardiovascular diseases and
enhanced activity of renin-angiotensin system in
psoriatic patients. *Acta Cardiologica* **40**: 199–205.

[4] Henseler T, Christophers E (1995). Disease
concomitance in psoriasis. *Journal of the American
Academy of Dermatology* **32**: 982–986.

[5] Mallbris L, Akre O, Granath F, *et al.* (2004).
Increased risk for cardiovascular mortality in
psoriasis inpatients but not in outpatients.
European Journal of Epidemiology **19**: 225–230.

[6] Gelfand JM, Neimann AL, Shin DB, *et al.* (2006).
Risk of myocardial infarction in patients with
psoriasis. *Journal of the American Medical
Association* **296**: 1735–1741.

[7] Peckham PE, Weinstein GD, McCullough JL
(1987). The treatment of severe psoriasis.
A national survey. *Archives of Dermatology*
123: 1303–1307.

[8] Wakkee M, Thio HB, Prens EP, *et al.* (2007).
Unfavorable cardiovascular risk profiles in
untreated and treated psoriasis patients.
Atherosclerosis **190**: 1–9.

[9] Maradit-Kremers H, Crowson CS, Nicola PJ, *et al.*
(2005). Increased unrecognized coronary heart
disease and sudden deaths in rheumatoid
arthritis: A population-based cohort study.
Arthritis and Rheumatism **52**: 402–411.

[10] Maradit-Kremers H, Nicola PJ, Crowson CS, *et al.*
(2005). Cardiovascular death in rheumatoid
arthritis: A population-based study. *Arthritis and
Rheumatism* **52**: 722–732.

[11] Ridker PM, Libber P (2005). Risk factors for
atherothrombotic disease. In: *Braunwald's Heart
Disease: A Textbook of Cardiovascular Medicine*, 7th
edn. DP Zipes (ed.). Saunders, Philadelphia.

[12] Sommer DM, Jenisch S, Suchan M, *et al.* (2006).
Increased prevalence of the metabolic syndrome
in patients with moderate to severe psoriasis.
Archives of Dermatological Research **298**: 321–328.

[13] Neimann AL, Shin DB, Wang X, *et al.* (2006).
Prevalence of cardiovascular risk factors in
patients with psoriasis. *Journal of the American
Academy of Dermatology* **55**: 829–835.

[14] Gisondi P, Tessari G, Conti A, *et al.* (2007).
Prevalence of metabolic syndrome in patients
with psoriasis: A hospital-based case-control
study. *British Journal of Dermatology* **157**: 68–73.

[15] Kremers HM, McEvoy MT, Dann FJ, Gabriel SE
(2007). Heart disease in psoriasis. *Journal of the
American Academy of Dermatology* **57**: 347–354.

[16] Isomaa B, Almgren P, Tuomi T, *et al.* (2001).
Cardiovascular morbidity and mortality associated with the metabolic syndrome. *Diabetes Care*
24: 693–699.

[17] Expert Panel on Detection, Evaluation, and
Treatment of High Blood Cholesterol in Adults
(2001). Executive summary of the third report of
the National Cholesterol Education Program
(NCEP) (Adult Treatment Panel III). *Journal of the
American Medical Association* **285**: 2486–2497.

[18] Balkau B, Vernay M, Mhamdi L, *et al.* (2003).
The incidence and persistence of the NCEP
(National Cholesterol Education Program)
metabolic syndrome. The French D.E.S.I.R.
study. *Diabetes and Metabolism* **29**: 526–532.

[19] Sattar N, Gaw A, Scherbakova O, *et al.* (2003).
Metabolic syndrome with and without C-reactive
protein as a predictor of coronary heart disease
and diabetes in the West of Scotland Coronary
Prevention Study. *Circulation* **108**: 414–419.

[20] Villegas R, Perry IJ, Creagh D, *et al.* (2003).
Prevalance of the metabolic syndrome in middle-
aged men and women. *Diabetes Care*
26: 3198–3199.

[21]   Lakksonen DE, Lakka HM, Niskanen LK, *et al.* (2002). Metabolic syndrome and development of diabetes mellitus: An application and validation of recently suggested definitions of the metabolic syndrome in a prospective cohort study. *American Journal of Epidemiology* **156**: 1070–1077.

[22]   Ford ES, Giles WH, Dietz WH (2002). Prevalence of the metabolic syndrome among U.S. adults: Findings from the Third National Health and Nutrition Examination Survey. *Journal of the American Medical Association* **287**: 356–359.

[23]   Cameron AJ, Shaw JE, Zimmet PZ (2004). The metabolic syndrome: Prevalence in worldwide populations. *Endocrinology and Metabolism Clinics* **33**: 2.

[24]   Mallbris L, Granath F, Hamsten A, Ståhle M (2006). Psoriasis is associated with lipid abnormalities at the onset of skin disease. *Journal of the American Academy of Dermatology* **54**: 614–621.

[25]   Sterry W, Strober BE, Menter A (2007). Obesity in psoriasis: The metabolic, clinical, and therapeutic implications. Report of an interdisciplinary conference and review. *British Journal of Dermatology* **157**: 649–655.

[26]   Reid AE (2006). Nonalcoholic fatty liver disease. In: *Feldman: Sleisenger and Fordtran's Gastrointestinal and Liver Disease*, 8th edn. M Feldman, LS Friedman, LJ Brandt (eds). Saunders, Philadelphia.

[27]   Whiting-O'Keefe QE, Fyfe KH, Sack KD (1991). Methotrexate and histologic hepatic abnormalities: A meta-analysis. *American Journal of Medicine* **90**: 711–716.

[28]   Saporito FC, Menter MA (2004). Methotrexate and psoriasis in the era of new biologic agents. *Journal of the American Academy of Dermatology* **50**: 301–309.

[29]   Teoh NC, Farrell GC. Drug-induced steatohepatitis, hepatic fibrosis, and cirrhosis. In: *Feldman: Sleisenger and Fordtran's Gastrointestinal and Liver Disease*, 8th edn. M Feldman, LS Friedman, LJ Brandt (eds). Saunders, Philadelphia.

[30]   Saadeh S, Younossi Z, Remer I, *et al.* (2002). The utility of radiological imaging in nonalcoholic fatty liver disease. *Gastroenterology* **123**: 745–750.

[31]   Becker U, Dies A, Sorensen TI, *et al.* (1996). Prediction of risk of liver disease by alcohol intake, sex and age: A prospective population study. *Hepatology* **23**: 1025–1029.

[32]   Chaput JC, Poynard T, Naveau S, *et al.* (1985). Psoriasis, alcohol, and liver disease. *British Medical Journal* **291**: 25.

[33]   Strange S, Dorn J, Muti P, *et al.* (2004). Body fat distribution, relative weight, and liver enzyme levels: A population-based study. *Hepatology* **39**: 754–763.

[34]   El-Serag H, Tran I, Everhart J (2004). Diabetes increases risk of chronic liver disease and hepatocellular carcinoma. *Gastroenterology* **126**: 460–468.

[35]   Edmundson WF, Guy WB (1958). Treatment of psoriasis with folic acid antagonist. *Archives of Dermatology* **78**: 200–203.

[36]   Bergstresser PR, Schreiber SH, Weinstein GD (1976). Systemic chemotherapy for psoriasis: A national survey. *Archives of Dermatology* **112**: 977–981.

[37]   Weinstein G, Roegnik H, Maibach H, *et al.* (1973). Cooperative study, psoriasis–liver–methotrexate interactions. *Archives of Dermatology* **108**: 36–42.

[38]   Malatjalian DA (1996). Methotrexate hepatotoxicity in psoriatics: Report of 104 patients from Nova Scotia, with analysis of risks from obesity, diabetes, and alcohol consumption during long term follow up. *Canadian Journal of Gastroenterology* **10**: 369–375.

[39]   Zachariae H, Kragballe K, Søgaard H (1980). Methotrexate induced liver cirrhosis. Studies including serial liver biopsies during continued tretment. *British Journal of Dermatology* **102**: 407–412.

[40]   Nyfors A (1977). Liver biopsies from psoriatics related to methotrexate therapy. 3. Findings in post-methotrexate liver biopsies from 160 psoriatics. *Acta Pathologica et Microbiologica Scandinavica* **85**: 511–518.

[41]   Thomas JA, Aithal GP (2005). Monitoring liver function during methotrexate therapy for psoriasis: Are routine biopsies really necessary? *American Journal of Clinical Dermatology* **6**: 357–363.

[42] Erickson A, Reddy V, Vogelgesang S, West S (1995). Usefulness of the American College of Rheumatology recommendations for liver biopsy in methotrexate-treated rheumatoid arthritis patients. *Arthritis and Rheumatism* **38**: 1115–1119.

[43] Zachariae H, Søgaard H (1987). Methotrexate-induced liver cirrhosis, a follow-up. *Dermatologica* **175**: 178–182.

[44] Zachariae H, Søgaard H, Heickendorff L (1996). Methotrexate-induced liver cirrhosis, clinical, histological and serological studies – a further 10-year follow-up. *Dermatology* **192**: 343–346.

[45] Carneiro SC, Cassia FF, Lamy F, *et al.* (2008). Methotrexate and liver function: A study of 13 psoriasis cases treated with different cumulative dosages. *Journal of the European Academy of Dermatology and Venereology* **22**: 25–29.

[46] Henning JS, Gruson LM, Strober BE (2007). Reconsidering liver biopsies during methotrexate therapy. *Journal of the American Academy of Dermatology* **56**: 893–894.

[47] Menter A, Korman NJ, Elmets CA, *et al.* (2009). Guidelines of care for the management of psoriasis and psoriatic arthritis: Section 4. Guidelines for the management and treatment of psoriasis with traditional systemic agents. *Journal of the American Academy of Dermatology* **61(3)**: 451–485.

[48] Pathirana D, Ormerod A, Saiag P, *et al.* (2009). European S3-Guidelines on the systemic treatment of psoriasis vulgaris. *Journal of the European Academy of Dermatology and Venereology* **2(23)**: 1–70.

[49] Chalmers R.J., Kirby B., Smith A., Burrows P., Little R., Horan M., *et al.* (2005). Replacement of routine liver biopsy by procollagen III amino-peptide for monitoring patients with psoriasis receiving long-term methotrexate: a multicenter audit and health economic analysis. *British Journal of Dermatology* **152**: 444–450.

[50] Laharie D (2006). Diagnosis of liver fibrosis by transient elastography (FibroScan) and non-invasive methods in Crohn's disease patients treated with methotrexate. *Alimentary Pharmacology and Therapeutics* **23**: 1621–1628.

[51] Griffiths CEM, Barker JNWN (2007). Psoriasis: Pathogenesis and clinical features. *Lancet* **370**: 263–271.

[52] Ho P, Bruce IN, Silman A, *et al.* (2005). Evidence for common genetic control in pathways of inflammation for Crohn's disease and psoriatic arthritis. *Arthritis and Rheumatism* **52**: 3596–3602.

[53] Bernstein CN, Wajda A, Blanchard JF (2005). The clustering of other chronic inflammatory diseases in inflammatory bowel disease: A population-based study. *Gastroenterology* **129**: 827–836.

[54] Lee FI, Bellary SV, Francis C (1990). Increased occurrence of psoriasis in patients with Crohn's disease and their relatives. *American Journal of Gastroenterology* **85**: 962–963.

[55] Plant D, Lear J, Marsland A, *et al.* (2004). CARD15/NOD2 single nucleotide polymorphisms do not confer susceptibility to type 1 psoriasis. *British Journal of Dermatology* **151**: 675–678.

[56] Najarian DJ, Gottlieb AB (2003). Connections between psoriasis and Crohn's disease. *Journal of the American Academy of Dermatology* **48**: 805–821.

[57] Sukal SA, Nadaminti L, Granstein RD (2006). Etanercept and demyelinating disease in a patient with psoriasis. *Journal of the American Academy of Dermatology* **54**:160–164.

[58] Enbrel (2005). Package insert. Immunex, Thousand Oaks, CA.

[59] Yamauchi PS, Gindi V, Lowe NJ (2004). The treatment of psoriasis and psoriatic arthritis with etanercept: Practical considerations on monotherapy, combination therapy and safety. *Dermatologic Clinics* **22**: 449–459, ix.

[60] Tauber WB. Serious adverse effects associated with the use of anti-TNF alpha drugs. Available from: www.fda.gov/cder/present/DIA2004/Tauber_files/frame.htm (accessed July 2005).

[61] Cisternas M, Gutierrez M, Jacobelli S (2002). Successful rechallenge with anti-tumor necrosis factor alpha for psoriatic arthritis after development of demyelinating nervous system disease during initial treatment: Comment on the article by Mohan *et al. Arthritis and Rheumatism* **46**: 3107–3108.

[62] Annuziata P, Morana P, Giorgia A, *et al.* (2003). High frequency of psoriasis in relatives is associated with early onset in an Italian multiple sclerosis cohort. *Acta Neurologica Scandinavica* **108**: 327–331.

[63] Methotrexate (2002). Package insert. Bedford Laboratories, Bedford, OH.

[64] Neoral (1995). Package insert. Sandoz Pharmaceuticals, Holzkirchen.

[65] Stern RS (2006). Lymphoma risk in psoriasis: Results of the PUVA follow-up study. *Archives of Dermatology* **142**: 1132–1135.

[66] Gelfand JM, Shin DB (2006). The risk of lymphoma in patients with psoriasis. *Journal of Investigative Dermatology* **126**: 2194–2201.

[67] Esposito M, Saraceno R, Giunta A, *et al.* (2006). An Italian study on psoriasis and depression. *Dermatology* **212**: 123–127.

[68] Gupta MA, Schork NJ, Gupta AK, *et al.* (1993). Suicidal ideation in psoriasis. *International Journal of Dermatology* **32**: 188–190.

[69] Richards HL, Fortune DG, Weidmann A, *et al.* (2004). Detection of psychological distress in patients with psoriasis: Low consensus between dermatologist and patient. *British Journal of Dermatology* **151**: 1227–1233.

[70] Lindegard B (1986). Diseases associated with psoriasis in the general population of 159,200 middle-aged, urban native Swedes. *Dermatologica* **172**: 298–304.

[71] Morse RM, Perry HO, Hurt RD (1985). Alcoholism and psoriasis. *Alcoholism, Clinical and Experimental Research* **9**: 396–399.

[72] Higgins EM, Peters TJ, du Vivier AM (1993). Smoking, drinking, and psoriasis. *British Journal of Dermatology* **129**: 749–750.

[73] Poikolainen K, Reunala T, Karvonen J, *et al.* (1990). Alcohol intake: A risk factor for psoriasis in young and middle-aged men. *British Journal of Medicine* **300**: 780–783.

[74] Poikolainen K, Reunula T, Karvonen J (1994). Smoking, alcohol and life events related to psoriasis among women. *British Journal of Dermatology* **130**: 473–477.

[75] Gelfand JM, Troxel AB, Lewis JD, *et al.* (2007). The risk of mortality in patients with psoriasis: Results from a population-based study. *Archives of Dermatology* **143**: 1493–1499.

CLINICIAN AND PATIENT RESOURCES

American Academy of Dermatology
(www.aad.org)

British Association of Dermatologists
(www.bad.org.uk)

British Skin Foundation
(www.britishskinfoundation.org)

European Academy of Venereology and Dermatology
(www.eadv.com)

International Psoriasis Council
(www.psoriasiscouncil.org)

National Psoriasis Foundation
(www.psoriasis.org)

The Psoriasis Association
(www.psoriasis-association.org.uk)

INDEX

Note: Page references in *italic* refer to tables or boxes in the text

A

ACCEPT trial 113
acitretin 96–97, *109*
acneiform eruption 83
ACR response criteria for rheumatoid arthritis (ACR-20) 118, 127
  applications 103, 106
acro-osteolysis 76, *80*
acrodermatitis continua of Hallopeau 26, 49
adalimumab 99, 102–103, 111, 113
adhesion molecules 13, 18
African–Americans 11, *12*
age 11
alcohol consumption 93, *93*, 121, 123
alefacept 98, *99*, 100, 111
American Academy of Dermatology 93, 122
American College of Rheumatology 103, 118, 127
ankylosing spondylitis 73, 76, 80, *80*
annular psoriasis 70
anthralin (dithranol) 85
anti-IL-12p-40 antibody (ABT-874) 114
antigen-presenting cells (APCs) 13, *17*, 18–20
antigens, triggers of psoriasis 18, *19*
arthritis, *see* osteoarthritis; psoriatic arthritis; rheumatoid arthritis
arthritis mutilans 78, 79
aspergillosis *105*
assessment tools 28, 81, 125–134
athlete's foot (tinea pedis) 66–67
atopic dermatitis 57, 58–59
Auspitz, Heinrich 9
Auspitz sign 8, 9, 13
Australia *12*

B

balanitis 57, 68, 69
'bamboo spine' 76, 80, *80*
barbiturates *93*, 95
betamethasone dipropionate 84, *84*
bevacizumab 114
Biblical references to psoriasis 7
biologics 99–107
  benefits 98
  clinical trials 103, 106, 113–14
  combination therapy 111
  T-cell modulators 98–101, *99*, 111
  TNF-a inhibitors *99*, 101–104, *105*, 110, 111, *111*, 113, *113*
body surface area measurement (BSA) 81
bone marrow suppression 93

Bowen's disease 57, 70
buttocks 32, 48

C

C reactive protein (CRP) 76
calcineurin inhibitors 84, 114
calcipotriene 110
calcipotriol 84, *84*
calcitriol 84, *84*
cancer risk
  ciclosporin therapy 95
  PUVA therapy 90
Candida infections 57, 68–69
cardiovascular disease 104, 119–120
CASPAR criteria 79, *79*
CCHCR-1, *see* coiled-coil α-helical rod protein 1
CD4+ cells, *see* T cells, CD4+
CD8+ cells, *see* T cells, CD8+
Celsus, Aurelius 7
cephalosporins 93
CHAMPION study 92, 113
China *12*
chromosome, defined *14*
chromosome 1 16
chromosome 3 16
chromosome 6 15
chromosome 17 15, 74
ciclosporin 94–95
  combination therapy *109*, 110
  dosing and monitoring 94
  interactions 95
  rotation therapy *111*
  sequential therapy 112
  side effects 95
cigarette smoking 120
cirrhosis 122
clinical trials
  biologics 103, 106, 113–114
  methotrexate 92, 113
coal tar preparations 45, 85, 108
coccidioidomycosis *105*
coiled-coil α-helical rod protein 1 (CCHCR-1) 15
colchicine *93*
corneodesmosin (CDSN) 15
corticosteroids
  topical 82–83, 84, *84*, 108
  withdrawal of oral 26
Croatia *12*, 73
Crohn's disease 16, 110, 122
cryptococcal infections *105*
cutaneous lymphocyte antigen (CLA) 13
cutaneous T-cell lymphoma (CTCL) 57, 70–71, 123
CXC-chemokine receptor 3 (CXCR3) 17
cytokines 12, 17, 20, 21–23, 113
  inhibitors/antagonists 113–114, *113*

D

dactylitis 74, 75, *80*
De re medica (Celsus) 7
demyelination neurological disease 104, *105*
dendritic cells (DCs) 18, 19
  dermal 19, 21
  plasmacytoid 20
depressive disorders 116, 123
dermatitis (eczema) 57, 58–60
Dermatology Life Quality Index (DLQI) 105, 117, 134
dermatophyte infections 64–67
dermis, histological changes 12–13
desmosomes 13
diabetes mellitus 66, 120–121
dilantin *93*
dimethylfumarate 97
distal interphalangeal (DIP) joints 76, 77
dithranol 85
drug development 113–114
drug interactions *93*, 95

E

E-cadherin 13
E-selectin 13, 18, 21
ears 35
eczema (dermatitis) 57, 58–60
efalizumab *99*, 100–101
elbows 30, 31
enthesitis 74, 75, *80*
epidemiology 11–12
epidermal histology 13–14
erythrocyte sedimentation rate 76
erythrodermic psoriasis 26, 44–45
erythromycins 95
etanercept *99*, 101–102, 111, *111*, 113
ethnicity 11
European Academy of Dermatology and Venereology 122
extensor surfaces 25

F

facial psoriasis 32–33
Faroe Islands *12*
feet
  nonpustular psoriasis 26, 40–41, 67
  pustular psoriasis 46–47
  tinea infections 57, 66–67
flexural disease 25, 37–8
follicular psoriasis 28, 52
France 73
fumaric acid esters 97

G

Galen 7
gastrointestinal disease 121–122
gender 11, 74, *80*
gene, defined *14*

genetics 14–16, 113, 114
    psoriatic arthritis 74
genital areas
    candidal infections 57, 68–69
    psoriasis 38
'geographic' forms 53
'geographic' tongue 34
geographical distribution of psoriasis
    12, 12
Germany 120
Goeckerman therapy 9, 45, 88, 108
Goeckerman, William 9
granulomatous infections 104, 105
groin disease 66
growth factors, antagonists 114
guttate psoriasis 26, 43, 61, 69

H
hands
    nonpustular psoriasis 26, 42
    pityriasis rubra pilaris 62, 63
    psoriatic arthritis 76–79
    pustular psoriasis 48
    see also nail disease
Health Assessment Questionnaire
    (HAQ) 116–117, 132–133
health-related quality of life (HRQOL)
    92
    assessment tools 81, *81*, 116–118,
    126–134
    and biologic therapy 103
    impact of psoriasis 115–116, *115*
Heberden's nodes 79
Hebra, Ferdinand 7–8
hepatic fibrosis 121, 122
hepatic toxicity
    methotrexate therapy 93, *93*, 121,
    122
    TNF-α inhibitors 104, 105
hepatitis B, screening 104
'herald patch' 60
high density lipoprotein (HDL) 121
Hippocrates 7
histological changes 12–14
histoplasmosis *105*
history of psoriasis 7–10, *9*
HIV-AIDS 66
HLA alleles, *see* human leucocyte
    antigen (HLA) alleles
Hodgkin's disease 123
human leucocyte antigen (HLA) alleles
    15, 74
hydroxyurea 97
hypercalcemia, secondary 84
hyperkeratosis, subungual 28, 51
hyperlipidemia 120–121

I
IFN-γ, *see* interferon-γ
IL, *see* interleukin
immunoglobulins 74
immunopathogenesis 16–24, 74

immunosuppressive therapy 66, 95
impact of disease 115–116
incidence of psoriasis 11
India *12*
infectious disease
    mimicking psoriasis 64–67
    and TNF-α inhibitor therapy 104,
    105
inflammatory bowel disease 73
inflammatory skin disease, mimicking
    psoriasis 57, 58–63
inflammatory (unstable) psoriasis 28,
    54–55
infliximab *99*, 103–104, 111
infusion-related problems 104
Ingram regimen 88
inheritance patterns 14
integrin 13
intercellular adhesion molecule-1
    (ICAM-1) 21
interferon-γ (IFN-γ) 17, 20, 22–23
interleukin-8 (IL-8) 21, 22
interleukin-10 (IL-10) 22
interleukin-12 (IL-12) 20, 22
    inhibitors 106–7
interleukin-17 (IL-17) 17, 20, 22–23
interleukin-22 (IL-22) 18, 20, 22–23
interleukin-23 (IL-23) 17–18, 20, 23,
    106
    inhibitors 106–107
International Psoriasis Council 81, 121,
    124
intertriginous areas 25
ISA-247 114
Italy *12*

J
joint stiffness, morning 74, 80

K
keratinocytes, proliferation 12, 13, 21
ketoconazole 95
Koebner, Heinrich 9, 114
Koebner phenomenon 8, 9, 20, 28, 56
Kogoj, spongiform pustules 13, 21
Koo Dr J. 112
Koo–Menter Psoriasis Instrument 92,
    117–118, 128–129

L
Langerhans cells 19
laser therapy 114
'lepra' 7
LFA-1, *see* lymphocyte function-
    associated antigen 1
linkage analysis *14*, 74
liver biopsy 94, 122
liver disease, *see* hepatic fibrosis; hepatic
    toxicity
LL37 20

locus (loci)
    associated with psoriasis 15–16
    defined 14, *14*
lymphocyte function-associated antigen
    1 (LFA-1) 17
lymphoma
    cutaneous T-cell (CTCL) 57, 70–71,
    123
    risk and PUVA therapy 123
    risk and TNF-α inhibitors 104, *105*
lysosomal-associated membrane protein
    (LAMP) 19

M
macrophages 24
major histocompatibility complex
    (MHC) *14*, 18–19
Mayo Clinic 11
measurement of disease 28, 81,
    125–134
metabolic syndrome 120–121, *120*
metacarpal-phalangeal (MCP) joints
    76, 77
methotrexate 92 4
    clinical trial 92, 113
    combination therapy 103–104,
    109, 110, *110*
    contraindications 93, *93*
    interactions 93
    liver biopsies 94, 122
    mode of action 92
    rotation therapy *111*
    sequential therapy 112
    side effects and toxicity 93, *93*, 121,
    122
MI, *see* myocardial infarction
mimics of psoriasis 57, *57*
    infectious skin disease 64–69
    inflammatory skin disease 58–63
    neoplasia 70–71
Moll and Wright classification 76, *76*
monocytes 24
monoethylfumarate 97
mortality 124
multiple sclerosis 104, 123
Munro microabscesses 13, 21
Munro, W.J. 9
mycobacterial infections, atypical *105*
mycophenolate mofetil 97
mycosis fungoides 70
myocardial infarction 119–120

N
nail disease
    pitting 50
    pityriasis rubra pilaris 62
    psoriasis 26, 28, 50, 51, 67
    psoriatic arthritis 74, 75, *80*
    tinea unguium 66–67
NAT9 (N-acetyltransferase 9) gene 15
National Psoriasis Foundation 115, 116
natural killer (NKT) cells 13, 16, 17

neck 34
neoplasms 57, 70–71
neurological disease 104, *105*
neutrophils 24
NF-AT, *see* nuclear factor of activated T cell (NF-AT)
NFκB, *see* nuclear factor-κB
NHERF1 gene 15
nitric oxide synthase, inducible (iNOS) 106
non-steroidal anti-inflammatory drugs (NSAIDs) *93*, 95, 112
nonpustular psoriasis (plaque type) 25–26
    generalized 26, 43–45
    localized 25–26, 30–42
Norway *12*, 73
nuclear factor of activated T cell (NF-AT) 114
nuclear factor-κB (NFκB) 20
nucleotide, defined *14*
nummular eczema *57*, 59

O
obesity 120, *121*
'oil drops' 26, *51*
oligoarthritis, asymmetric 76, *76*, 77
onycholysis 26, *51*
onychomycosis 66
oral disease 34
osteoarthritis 79, *80*
osteopenia, juxta-articular 76
osteophytes 79, *80*
Outcome Measures in Rheumatoid Arthritis Clinical Trials (OMERACT) 118

P
palmoplantar psoriasis
    efalizumab therapy 100, *101*
    nonpustular 26, 40–42
    pustular 26, 46–48, 60
parakeratosis 13
PASI, *see* Psoriasis Area and Severity Index
pathogenesis 12
    common to psoriasis and MI 119
    genetics 14–16
    immunology 16–24
    psoriatic arthritis 21, 74
'pencil in cup' deformity 76
penicillins *93*
periodic-acid Schiff (PAS) 65
pharmacogenomics 114
PHOENIX I and II trials 106
phototherapy 86–89
    broadband UVB 86–87, *87*
    combination 88, 96, 109–110, *109*
    narrowband 87
    rotation therapy *111*
    targeted 88–89

    see also psoralen with ultraviolet A (PUVA) therapy
physical impairment 115
Physician's Global Assessment (PGA) 125
pimecrolimus 84
pityriasis rosea *57*, 60–61
pityriasis rubra pilaris *57*, 62–63
plaque-type psoriasis, *see* nonpustular psoriasis
plaques 25–26
    discoid 25
    large 28, 53
    small 28, 52
polyarthritis, symmetric 77
potassium hydroxide (KOH) 65, 66
prevalence of psoriasis 11
probenecid *93*, 95
procollagen IIIA test *93*, 122
'pseudohyphae' 68
psoralen with ultraviolet A (PUVA) therapy 71, 89–90
    cautions and contraindications 90
    combination therapies 88, 96, 109–110
    lymphoma risk 123
    rotation therapy *111*
    sequential 112
Psoriasis Area and Severity Index (PASI) 28, 81, 125
    and biologic therapy 102, 103
Psoriasis Disability Index (PDI) 126–127
psoriatic arthritis 73
    assessment tools 118, 127
    biologic therapy 103, 106
    clinical manifestations 74–80
    diagnostic criteria 79, *79*
    differential diagnosis 79–80, *80*
    epidemiology 73–74
    genetics and pathogenesis 15, 21, 74
    onset in psoriasis 73–74
    prognosis 80
    subtypes 76–79, *76*
Psoriatic Arthritis-specific Quality of Life instrument (PsAQoL) 118, 127
PSORS1 locus 15, 74
PSORS2 locus 15, 74
PSORS4 locus 16
PSORS5 locus 16
PSORS6–10 loci 16
psychiatric disorders 123
psychosocial impairment 116
pulse therapy 84
pulsed-dye laser 114
purified protein derivative (PPD) test *105*
purpura 83

pustular psoriasis 26
    generalized (von Zumbusch type) 26, 50
    histology 13
    localized 46–49
PUVA, *see* psoralen with ultraviolet A (PUVA) therapy

Q
quality of life, *see* health-related quality of life (HRQOL)

R
race 11
RAPTOR gene 15
Reiter syndrome 73
renal function, ciclosporin therapy 95
rete ridges 13
retinoids
    combination therapy 88, 96, *109*, 110, *110*
    sequential therapy 112
    side effects 97
    systemic 96–97
    topical 85, 88
rheumatoid arthritis (RA) 79, *80*, 110
    assessment tools 118, 127
rheumatoid factor (RF) 73, 79, *80*
RUNX1 15

S
sacroiliitis 76, *80*
Salford Psoriasis Index 117
Samoa *12*
scale 25, 60, 61
scalp disease
    psoriasis 26, 39–40, 64
    tinea capitis 64
scar sites 56
'sebo-psoriasis' 25, 36
self-DNA 20
Sézary syndrome 70, 71
Short Form 36 (SF-36) 116, 130–131
signal transducer and activator of transcription 1 (STAT 1) 20, 22
single nucleotide polymorphisms (SNPs) *14*, 15, 74
SLC9A3R1 gene 15
smoking 120
socioeconomic status 115
South America *12*
spine, psoriatic arthritis 76, *80*
spondyloarthropathies, 'seronegative' 73
spongiform pustules of Kogoj 13, 21
squamous cell carcinoma *in situ* (Bowen's disease) *57*, 70
stable *vs* unstable disease 28, 54–56
Stanford Health Assessment Questionnaire (HAQ) 116–117, 132–133

steatohepatitis 121
streptococcal infections 26
striae 83
subungual hyperkeratosis 28, 51
suicidal ideation 116, 123
sulfonamides 93, 95
Sweden 12, 73
syndesmophytes 76, 80
syndrome X, *see* metabolic syndrome
syphilis, secondary 57, 68–69

T
T cells 13, 16–18
    antibodies 114
    CD4+ (helper) 13, 17, 17, 22–23,
    100
    CD8+ 13, 17, 17
    CD11c+ 19
    natural killer (NKT) 17
T-cell modulating agents 98–101, 99,
    111
tacalcitol 84, 84
tachyphylaxis 83
tacrolimus 84
tar-based therapy 45, 85, 108
tazarotene, topical 85
telangiectases 83
therapy 81
    biologics 99–107
    combination 108–112
    future developments 113–114
    phototherapy and PUVA 86–90
    rationale for systemic 91–92, 91
    rotational 111, 111
    sequential 112, 112
    topical 82–85
    traditional systemic agents 91–97
    undertreatment 92
6-thioguanine 97
thymidylate synthetase 114
tinea infections 57, 64–67
toll-like receptors (TLR) 20, 23
tongue 34
transforming growth factor-α (TGF-α)
    21
transient elastography 122
Trichophyton rubrum 65, 66
Trichophyton tonsurans 64
triggers of psoriasis 18, 19
trimethoprim 95
tuberculosis 104, 105
tumor necrosis factor-α (TNF-α) 21–22
    drugs targeting 22, 99, 101–104,
    105, 110, 111, 111, 113, 113
twin studies 14, 74

U
ultraviolet light therapy, *see*
    phototherapy; psoralen with ultra-
    violet A (PUVA) therapy
umbilicus 31
undertreatment 92
United Kingdom 12
United States 12, 73
ustekinumab 99, 106–107, 113

V
vascular adhesion molecule 1 (VCAM-1)
    21
vascular endothelial growth factor
    (VEGF) 13, 106
    antagonists 114
very low density lipoprotein (VDL) 121
vitamin D3 derivatives 84
von Zumbusch, Leo 10
'von Zumbusch type' psoriasis 26, 50

W
Willan, Robert 7
Woronoff, D.L. 10
Woronoff's ring 10